Nutrition and Neurodisability

T0178907

Nutrition and Neurodisability

Edited by
Peter B Sullivan
MA MD FRCP FRCPCH, Emeritus Professor in Paediatric Gastroenterology;
Associate Dean (Postgraduate Medicine), Medical Sciences Division
University of Oxford, Oxford, UK

Guro L Andersen
Senior Consultant Habilitation Center and leader of the Cerebral Palsy
Registry of Norway; Associate Professor, Department of Clinical
and Molecular Medicine, Faculty of Medicine and Health Sciences
Norwegian University of Science and Technology, Trondheim, Norway

Morag J Andrew
Consultant in Community Paediatrics, Department of Paediatrics,
The Great North Children's Hospital, Newcastle Upon Tyne, UK

2020
Mac Keith Press

© 2020 Mac Keith Press

Managing Director: Ann-Marie Halligan
Senior Publishing Manager: Sally Wilkinson
Publishing Co-ordinator: Lucy White
Project Management: Riverside Publishing Solutions Ltd

First published in this edition in 2020 by Mac Keith Press
2nd Floor, Rankin Building, 139–143 Bermondsey Street, London, SE1 3UW

British Library Cataloguing-in-Publication data
A catalogue record for this book is available from the British Library

Cover designer: Marten Sealby

ISBN: 978-1-911612-25-4

Typeset by Riverside Publishing Solutions Ltd
Printed by Hobbs the Printers Ltd, Totton, Hampshire, UK

Contents

Contents

Author
Appointments

Guro L Andersen Senior Consultant Habilitation Center and leader of the Cerebral Palsy Registry of Norway; Associate Professor, Department of Clinical and Molecular Medicine, Faculty of Medicine and Health Sciences, Norwegian University of Science and Technology, Trondheim, Norway

Morag J Andrew Consultant in Community Paediatrics, Department of Paediatrics, The Great North Children's Hospital, Newcastle Upon Tyne, UK

Steven J Bachrach MD, Emeritus, Department of Pediatrics, Nemours/Al duPont Hospital for Children; Professor of Pediatrics, Sidney Kimmel Medical College of Thomas Jefferson University, Philadelphia, PA, USA

Kristie L Bell Accredited Practicing Dietitian, PhD, Dietetics and Food Services, Queensland Children's Hospital; Centre for Child Health Research, The University of Queensland, South Brisbane, Queensland, Australia

Katherine A Benfer Postdoctoral Research Fellow, Queensland Cerebral Palsy and Rehabilitation Research Centre, The University of Queensland, South Brisbane, Queensland, Australia

Ilse Broekaert Consultant Pediatric Gastroenterology, University of Cologne, Faculty of Medicine and University Hospital Cologne, Department of Pediatrics, Cologne, Germany

Isabelle Chase | Pediatric dentist with expertise in children with neurodevelopmental disabilities; Assistant Professor of Developmental Biology, Harvard School of Dental Medicine, Boston, MA, USA

Laurie Glader | Director, Complex Care Service Outpatient Program; Co-Director, Cerebral Palsy and Spasticity Center, Boston Children's Hospital; Assistant Professor of Pediatrics, Harvard Medical School, Boston, MA, USA

Jane Hardy | Associate Medical Director, Children's Community Health Service; Consultant Community Paediatrician, Community Paediatric Department, Manchester, UK

Amy Hughes | Assistant Professor, Department of Surgery, Division of Otolaryngology at Connecticut Children's Hospital, Hartford, CT, USA

Jessie M Hulst | Paediatric Gastroenterologist, PhD, Department of Paediatrics, Division of Gastoenterology, Hepatology and Nutrition, The Hospital for Sick Children; Assistant Professor of Paediatrics, University of Toronto, Toronto Ontario, Canada.

Heidi H Kecskemethy | Clinical Reseach Scientist, Department of Medical Imaging, Nemours Biomedical Research, Wilmington, DE, USA

Hayley Kuter | Paediatric Dietitian, Manchester University NHS Foundation Trust, Manchester, UK

Diane Sellers | Clinical Academic Speech and Language Therapist, Chailey Clinical Services, Sussex Community NHS Foundation Trust, North Chailey, East Sussex, UK

Peter B Sullivan | MA MD FRCP FRCPCH, Emeritus Professor in Paediatric Gastroenterology; Associate Dean (Postgraduate Medicine), Medical Sciences Division, University of Oxford, Oxford, UK

Jacqueline L Walker | Lecturer and Accredited Practicing Dietitian, PhD, School of Human Movement and Nutrition Sciences, The University of Queensland, St Lucia, Queensland, Australia

Kelly A Weir | Senior Lecturer, School of Allied Health Sciences & Menzies Health Institute Queensland, Griffith University Gold Coast Health, Southport, Queensland, Australia

Foreword

Enough and appropriate food and water are essential for human life. This statement is obvious. Nonetheless, lack of food, and starvation are regular occurring consequences of wars and natural disasters. During such crises, children, but also grown-ups, in particular elderly people, may die, or they become more vulnerable to other disorders, such as infectious diseases. In children, somatic growth and psychomotor development will be impaired.

In other settings where food is sufficient, meals are important elements in our social life, ranging from regular daily meals within the family, with friends or colleagues, to the most advanced tasting menus served in the best restaurants. In the short story, *Babette's feast*, the Danish author Karen Blixen, describes how Babette prepares an exquisite meal in a remote fishing village in Northern-Norway, using ingredients imported directly from Paris. Although the locals considered such a meal to be a sinful act, they felt how the meal lifted them both spiritually and physically, how local disagreement and anger evaporated, and love and peace settled on the table.

Persons with disabilities have a range of challenges related to feeding and nutrition. Among the most severe problems is severe oral-motor dysfunction. In early childhood, persons with such dysfunctions are at risk of being truly starved, and undernutrition may impair growth and neurodevelopment. Chewing and swallowing problems, and gastroesophageal reflux may lead to aspiration of food or gastric content into their airways, followed by pneumonia. The other extreme is overfeeding resulting in overweight and adiposity. The latter is often seen in some syndromes, such as Down syndrome and Prader Willi syndrome. However, a too high proportion of body fat may also be the result of misinterpretation of body composition in persons with disabilities where measures such as body mass index applied in the typical developing population may be misleading.

Ten years ago Mac Keith Press published the book *Feeding and nutrition in children with neurodevelopmental disability* edited by Peter Sullivan. That book became a recommended textbook for many professionals involved in the care for persons with neurodevelopmental disabilities. As Martin Bax stated in his foreword to that book, it was first towards the end of the 20th century that attention was paid to these problems.

This new book edited by Sullivan, Andersen and Andrews, includes the results of the most recent research and practical guidelines regarding assessment of feeding difficulties and body composition as well as the most recent recommendations regarding treatment. The authors of the various chapters are world-leading experts from Europe, Australia and North-America. The authors address all important aspects of this challenging topic. The practical perspective is essential and will certainly be appreciated by inter-professional teams trying to help optimizing the nutritional status of children and adults with disabilities.

In *Babette's feast* there were some original guests, but none with a clear neurodevelopmental disability. Within a family setting, severe feeding difficulties are likely to affect the family's quality of life. The application of the knowledge provided in this new book should provide a basis for enabling persons with disabilities to take part in, and enjoy any meal both in a private and a public setting, and even to experience such meals as presented in *Babette's feast*. Most importantly, the content in the book should contribute to a lighter daily life in families of persons with disabilities, and for the persons themselves.

Torstein Vik, Department of Clinical and Molecular Medicine,
Norwegian University of Science and Technology,
Trondheim, Norway

Preface

This book is the third produced on this topic by Mac Keith Press over the last three decades. Acknowledgement for this initiative should go to Martin Bax who as Editor of *Developmental Medicine & Child Neurology* realised that the nutritional needs of children with cerebral palsy were not adequately being met by health care professionals. The early texts on cerebral palsy make little or no mention of the feeding difficulties encountered in children with severe neurological impairment and feeding and nutritional assessment was not part of the routine care of these children. In the late 1980's, it was Martin who saw the advantage of teaming up a paediatric gastroenterologist with an interest in nutrition with a paediatric neurologist; this culminated in the first volume *Feeding the Disabled Child* edited by myself and Lewis Rosenbloom and published in 1996. Following Martin's retirement, Lewis, as Chair of the Editorial Board of Mac Keith Press persuaded me that an update in the form of a practical handbook was required. This lead to the publication of *Feeding and Nutrition in Children with Neurodevelopmental Disability* by Mac Keith Press in 2009. Now some ten years later and with increasing research interest and endeavour and with the appearance of guidelines from various learned bodies on the topic of nutritional and feeding problems in children with neurological impairment, Bernard Dan the current Editor in Chief of *Developmental Medicine & Child Neurology* considered it is necessary again to update the handbook.

This volume is designed to be a practical evidenced-based handbook aimed at health professionals who have responsibility for caring for children with the feeding, nutritional and gastrointestinal problems that ensue from neurological impairment and especially cerebral palsy. This book will be of value both for those new to this clinical field and for more experienced practitioners.

An appreciation of the development of the normal anatomy and physiology of the oral-motor apparatus is essential for understanding of the pathophysiology of oral-motor dysfunction that underlies the feeding problems in children with neurological impairment; these aspects are covered in the opening two chapters. Drooling of saliva is an important additional consequence of oral-motor dysfunction and this problem and its management is covered in a separate chapter. Oral-motor dysfunction is a component of an overall abnormality in gastrointestinal motility resulting in increased gastro-oesophageal reflux, delayed gastric emptying and constipation. Evaluation and management of these gastroenterological problems, which affect the great majority of children with neurological impairment and especially these children with cerebral palsy is covered in detail. Nutritional impairment is frequently a consequence of the feeding problems encountered by children with cerebral palsy and the impact of such undernutrition on growth, metabolism, cognitive and immune function may be overlooked. Recent research has led to a greater understanding of the adverse consequences of undernutrition and these are detailed in this volume.

Successful nutritional management depends upon accurate assessment and so the heart of this handbook comprises a series of chapters on assessment; these cover growth, energy balance, body composition, macro- and micronutrient intake, and dietetic assessment. Because children with neurodisabilities have risk for compromised bone health attributable to a combination of atypical muscle tone combined with lack of weight bearing resulting in reduced bone size and bone density, this new handbook devotes a whole chapter to this topic. All the assessment chapters describe the range of methods and techniques used in nutritional assessment together with an evaluation of the advantages and disadvantages of each technique and a discussion of the validity for their use in children with neurological impairment. The issue of (lack of) appropriate reference standards in children with neurological impairment for growth and nutritional intake is taken into account in the recommendations made.

Following on from detailed feeding, nutritional and gastroenterological assessment comes the development of a management strategy. Children with neurological impairment, and especially those with cerebral palsy, form a rather heterogeneous clinical group. Accordingly, management strategies must be individualised and targeted and the specific needs of each child. Furthermore, successful feeding, nutritional and gastroenterological management will not be the province of one particular professional discipline but will be the outcome of the input and endeavours of a multi-disciplinary team. These basic principles run through all the chapters on assessment and management. Where appropriate clinical case vignettes are used to illustrate points being made in the text and it is hoped that these will prove to be an instructive and valuable addition to the handbook.

Enteral tube feeding has transformed the landscape of nutritional management of children with cerebral palsy in recent years and whilst it circumvents the problems of feeding inefficiency and unsafe swallow associated with oral-motor impairment, the technique is not without its problems. Amongst these are included the complications of the procedure itself, the potential risk of overfeeding and the significant impact – both beneficial and adverse - that gastrostomy or jejunostomy tube feeding has on parents.

These issues are explored in detail in the penultimate chapter. The handbook ends with a resume of all the take home messages from each of the foregoing chapters.

In producing this handbook, the editors have sought contributions from the acknowledged leaders in each topic from around the world. It is our earnest hope that this handbook will prove to be a useful resource for any health professional engaged in the assessment and management of the feeding, nutritional and gastrointestinal problems in children with neurological impairment.

I would like to acknowledge the continuous help and support given to the editors to produce this handbook from Rosie Outred, Lucy White and Sally Wilkinson from Mac Keith Press.

Peter B Sullivan, Oxford
November 2019

CHAPTER 1

The Normal Development of Oral Motor Function: Anatomy and Physiology

Morag J Andrew

INTRODUCTION

An appreciation of the anatomy and physiology of normal feeding is helpful in considering feeding and swallowing difficulties which may arise in children with neurodisability. This chapter provides an overview of the normal anatomy, physiology and neuronal control of feeding, before considering the development of normal feeding in infancy and early childhood.

ANATOMY

Structural integrity of the mouth and pharynx are necessary for the development of normal eating and swallowing functions.

The pharynx is made up of three compartments: the nasopharynx, oropharynx and hypopharynx (Fig. 1.1). The nasopharynx is a muscular cavity whose anterior border is formed by the posterior nasal cavity at the level of the choana. The superior border is formed by the sphenoid sinus; the posterosuperior border by the clivus, upper cervical spine, and prevertebral muscles; and the inferior border by the soft palate. The nasopharynx contains the adenoids and communicates directly with the middle ear cavity via the eustachian tubes, sited in the lateral pharyngeal walls.

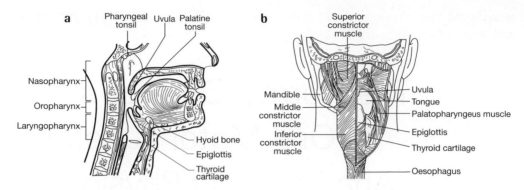

Figure 1.1 Anatomy of the oral cavity and pharynx. (Reprinted from Matsuo & Palmer 2008 with permission from Elsevier.)

The anterior border of the oropharynx is created by the circumvallate papillae of the tongue and the anterior tonsillar pillars, which separate the oropharynx from the oral cavity. Posteriorly the oropharynx is bound by the pharyngeal constrictor muscles and superiorly by the soft palate. Inferiorly it is separated from the larynx by the epiglottis and glossoepiglottic fold, and from the hypopharynx by the pharyngoepiglottic fold. It contains the tongue base, palatine tonsils, soft palate, and oropharyngeal mucosa and constrictor muscles from the level of the palate to the hyoid bone. The hypopharynx runs from the hyoid bone superiorly to the cricoid cartilage inferiorly. The hypopharynx begins at the inferior border of the oropharynx and connects with the cervical oesophagus at the cricopharyngeal muscle, which forms the upper oesophageal sphincter.

These three anatomic compartments have dual roles in the ingestion of liquids and foods and respiration. In order for feeding to proceed safely, careful coordination of these functions are required. Any disruption to the neural control of these mechanisms, for example following brain injury, may lead to aspiration of food or drink into the respiratory tract, with subsequent respiratory morbidity.

PHYSIOLOGY

Swallowing comprises of four phases: the oral preparatory, oral, pharyngeal and oesophageal phase. The first two phases are under voluntary control, with the pharyngeal phase being partly voluntary, but mostly involuntary, and the oesophageal phase entirely involuntary. For liquids, the oral preparatory phase requires containment and positioning of fluid within the oral cavity. The preparation of solids is more complex and involves the processing of food by the lips, teeth, cheeks and tongue to form a bolus. Food must be transported around the mouth to the teeth to be broken down into a more liquid state with the aid of saliva. Good lip seal, a coordinated range of tongue and jaw movements and normal oral sensation are all prerequisites for this phase to proceed effectively.

In the oral phase the food bolus is propelled backwards by elevation of the tongue with sequential contact between the hard and soft palates. When the bolus reaches the posterior oral cavity (e.g. soft palate and faucial pillars) the swallow reflex is initiated. This sensory stimulus on the posterior oral structures ends the voluntary oral phase and triggers the involuntary pharyngeal phase of the swallow.

During the pharyngeal phase, the velum elevates, closing off the nasopharynx, and the pharyngeal constrictors propel the bolus through the faucial pillars to the upper oesophageal sphincter (e.g. cricopharyngeus) in a peristaltic wave. At the same time, the larynx closes, elevates, and is pulled forward by the laryngeal strap muscles. The epiglottis and the aryepiglottic folds, the false vocal folds, and the true vocal folds form three separate levels of laryngeal closure, protecting the airway from penetration with food or liquid. Respiration stops briefly to allow the bolus to move to the relaxed upper oesophageal sphincter. The cricopharyngeus muscle functions as the valve at the top of the oesophagus. It remains in a fixed state of contraction and only relaxes to allow food or liquid to pass during a swallow.

The oesophageal phase then begins, continuing peristaltic transport of the bolus to the stomach.

The anatomy and physiology of swallowing is further reviewed by Sasegbon and Hamdy (2017).

NEURAL CONTROL OF EATING AND SWALLOWING

The neuroanatomy of swallowing is complex, but can be simplified into three categories: afferent neurons, interneurons and efferent neurons. Although individual cranial nerves may have a predominantly afferent or efferent role, most have both sensory and motor components.

Afferent Neurons

The afferent fibres of the trigeminal nerve (Cranial Nerve [CN] V) input sensory information from the mouth, whilst sensory information from the pharynx is provided by the facial (CN VII), glossopharyngeal (CN IX) and vagus (CN X) nerves. The superior laryngeal nerve is a branch of the vagus nerve and is formed from the inferior ganglion of the vagus nerve at the level of the second cervical vertebrae. It forms an external and internal branch at the level of the third cervical vertabrae. The external branch is predominantly a motor nerve and supplies the cricothyroid muscle, whilst the internal branch of the laryngeal nerve is largely sensory and supplies the pharynx and superior larynx. The facial nerve also supplies taste fibres to the anterior two thirds of the tongue and the glossopharyngeus nerve supplies taste fibres to the posterior third of the tongue.

These afferent neurons input to the nucleus tractus solitarius, a relay station in the medulla. The nucleus tractus solitarius communicates with swallowing neurons in the region of the nucleus ambiguous, which then drives the motor neurons and coordinates the complex sequence of muscle contraction required for effective oropharyngeal swallowing to occur. The network of coordinating neurons within the medulla oblongata is called the central pattern generator (CPG). Two CPGs exist, one on either side of the medulla oblongata; functionally they can be considered as a single unit. Each CPG is supplied by afferent nerve fibres from the ipsilateral side of the mouth and pharynx.

Interneurons

Interneurons synchronise communication between the two halves of the CPG. The CPG coordinates swallowing, but is mediated by subcortical and cortical inputs.

Efferent Neurons

The motor coordination of swallowing is controlled by the trigeminal (CN V), facial (CN VII), glossopharyngeal (CN IX), vagus (CN X), accessory (CN XI) and hypoglossal (CN XII) nerves. The trigeminal and hypoglossal nerves innervate most of the muscles of the oral cavity. The trigeminal nerve also innervates the muscles of mastication. The hypoglossal nerve innervates the intrinsic muscles of the tongue, whilst the extrinsic muscles, except for the palatoglossus (CN X) are innervated by the ansa cervicalis (C1–C2). The muscles of the palate, pharynx and larynx are predominantly innervated by the vagus nerve (CN X), with the exception of the tensor veli palatine in the soft palate, which is supplied by a subdivision of the mandibular branch of the trigeminal nerve (CN V).

Innervation of the Salivary Glands

There are three pairs of salivary glands: the parotid, submandibular and sublingual glands. These receive parasympathetic and sympathetic innervation. Parasympathetic drive increases salivary production, whilst sympathetic input makes saliva more viscous. The parotid salivary glands receive parasympathetic innervation from the glossopharyngeal nerve; the submandibular and sublingual glands receive parasympathetic innervation from the trigeminal nerve. Sympathetic fibres from the superior cervical ganglion inner-vate all three pairs of salivary glands.

For further information on the neural control of eating and swallowing, the reader is directed to Stevenson and Allaire (1996) and Sasegbon and Hamdy (2017).

THE NORMAL DEVELOPMENT OF EATING AND DRINKING SKILLS

It is helpful to consider feeding skills within a developmental context; as with all domains of childhood development, there is sequential progression of skills through infancy and early childhood in order to achieve competent and safe feeding. The development of normal feeding is a complex process and requires the integration of gross motor, fine motor, oral, communication and visual skills. Disruption to these processes may impact on the development of feeding and drinking skills; for example, failure to develop head control, sitting and truncal alignment is likely to compromise feeding position and swal-lowing safety unless external postural support is provided. Cognitive and behavioural development also impacts on the acquisition of feeding skills, as does the social and cultural context in which feeding is learnt.

In the newborn infant, rooting, latching, sucking and swallowing are entirely reflexive and are facilitated by the brainstem. Over the first 6 months of life the oral phase grad-ually moves from being under reflexive to volitional control, so that by the end of the first year feeding has changed from being a reflexive to a voluntary process (Stevenson & Allaire 1996). As with any developmental skill, refinement occurs through continual practice. In children with neurodisability, brainstem reflexes may persist leading to exaggerated or persistent primitive reflexes (e.g. tonic bite and gagging) which interfere with efficient feeding and drinking.

FEEDING DIFFICULTIES IN CHILDREN WITH NEURODISABILITY

Feeding difficulties are common in children with neurodisability, and are multifactorial. The causes of feeding difficulties in children with neurodisability are considered in detail in Chapter 2. Whilst this chapter has necessarily focused on body structure and function in the development of feeding skills, the following chapter considers feeding difficul-ties within the broader framework of The International Classification of Functioning, Disability and Health (WHO-ICF) (World Health Organization 2001). WHO-ICF is a classification of health and health-related domains linking body structures and func-tions, activity and participation, alongside health condition (disorder or disease) and contextual factors (personal and environmental). The ICF is WHO's framework for health and disability; it is the conceptual basis for the definition, measurement and policy for health and disability. As well as being important as a planning and policy tool for decision makers, it provides clinicians and researchers with a holistic approach to health and disability, and disability research.

REFERENCES

Matsuo K, Palmer JB (2008) Anatomy and physiology of feeding and swallowing – normal and abnormal. *Phys Med Rehabil Clin North Am* 19(4): 691–707.

Sasegbon A, Hamdy S (2017) The anatomy and physiology of normal and abnormal swallowing in oropharyngeal dysphagia. *Neurogastroenterol Motil* 29(11): e13100.

Stevenson RD, Allaire JH (1996) The development of eating skills in infants and young children. In: *Feeding the Disabled Child: Clinics in Developmental Medicine*, 1st edn. London: Mac Keith Press, pp. 11–22.

World Health Organization (2001) *International Classification of Functioning Disability and Health.* Geneva: World Health Organization.

CHAPTER 2

'When Things Go Wrong': Causes and Assessment of Oral Sensorimotor Dysfunction

Diane Sellers

INTRODUCTION

The previous chapter provides an outline of the anatomy and physiology of functional mechanisms of eating and swallowing. This chapter provides an overview of 'when things go wrong': the causes and consequences of disturbances to the movements required to ingest food and drink in cases of neurological impairment. A number of different disorders of the central nervous system in children may affect the movements required for safe and efficient eating and drinking, including cerebral palsy, acquired brain injury, genetic disorders and degenerative neurological disorders. Children born prematurely or with autistic spectrum disorder may present with eating and drinking challenges (Rommel et al. 2003; Thoyre et al. 2014); however, unless associated with some form of movement limitation, these difficulties are linked primarily to sensory and behavioural disturbances and will not be discussed here.

The movements of eating, drinking and swallowing require complex sensorimotor processes (Evans Morris & Dunn Klein 2001; Malandraki et al. 2011a; Crary 2016). Eating and drinking behaviours, including problematic ones, are likely to change over time because of the dynamic nature of these interacting and changing physiological systems linked to children's development, learning, experience and health.

Different approaches to clinical assessment of children's eating, drinking and swallowing difficulties associated with neurological impairments will be considered.

BODY FUNCTION, ACTIVITY AND PARTICIPATION

The International Classification of Functioning, Disability and Health (World Health Organization 2001) provides a unified framework representing the dynamic interactions between an individual and the environment. The concepts of **body function**, **activity**, **participation**, **personal factors** and **environmental factors** will be used to consider limitations to movements required for eating and drinking and swallowing, that is 'when things go wrong'.

Body Function: Movement and Posture

A child with a neurological disorder will find it challenging to control and coordinate muscle activity in the body. Muscles may be switched 'on', with higher tone than usual (hypertonia); children may be floppy with lower tone (hypotonia) or may experience a mixture of high, low and varying muscle tone. Other disturbances to movement come from muscle weakness. Skilled movement is also affected by reduced selective motor control (inability to recruit muscles with precision, speed or timing).

If postural stability is compromised by altered truncal muscle tone, finer movements required for eating, drinking and swallowing will be challenging. Postural assessment and management is an important aspect of the feeding assessment. Investigations carried out using dynamic X-ray filming (videofluoroscopy) have demonstrated the impact of changing head and trunk position on safety of swallow (Larnert & Ekberg 1995; Ertekin et al. 2001). In addition, some neurological disorders arising in childhood are accompanied by the retention of primitive reflexes, involuntary movements which also interfere with the development of skilled movements required for safe and efficient eating and drinking (Zafeiriou 2004). Postural management (Gericke 2006) may include special seating including head support suitable for mealtimes.

Whilst there is an association between gross motor ability and eating and drinking ability for children with cerebral palsy (Weir et al. 2013; Sellers et al. 2014a), some children will experience specific movement difficulties primarily affecting their eating, drinking and swallowing (Sullivan et al. 2002).

Body Function: Awareness, Sensation, Perception and Cognition

Motor disorders of neurological origin such as cerebral palsy are often accompanied by disturbances of sensation, perception, cognition, communication and behaviour (Rosenbaum et al. 2007). Epilepsy may be present having an overall impact on the individual's levels of arousal and awareness. Secondary musculoskeletal problems may also be present which are likely to be a source of pain (Ramstad et al. 2011). These additional disturbances will impact on eating and drinking performance.

The enjoyment and pleasure of eating and drinking comes from the integration of sensory information by the central nervous system: including the appearance, touch, taste, temperature, smell and sound of the food in the mouth (Spence 2015). Appetite, satiety, nausea and other feedback mechanisms from the gut also affect the enjoyment of feeding. The extent of an individual's sensory loss will not mirror the severity of motor deficit (Odding et al. 2006). The neurological disturbances of cerebral palsy will affect children's tactile sensory perception and integration and subsequent impact on function (Odding et al. 2006; Auld et al. 2012). Invasive or adverse events, such as nasogastric tube feeding in infancy, may also impact upon feeding because of long-term altered oral sensitivity and facial defensiveness (Dodrill et al. 2004).

A child's ability to respond automatically, efficiently and comfortably to eating and drinking experiences will be affected by disturbances to sensory processing which include altered registration of sensory input, excessive or low levels of reaction to sensation, limited sensory discrimination, difficulty integrating information and difficulty planning motor responses.

Functional MRI studies and instrumental measures provide some insights into essential sensory perception and processing linked to eating, drinking and swallowing with major implications for safety as well as function and enjoyment (Malandraki et al. 2011a, b; Ulualp et al. 2013).

Body Function: Breathing, Eating, Drinking and Swallowing

Having outlined potential issues linked to the whole body, it is important to consider the detailed component parts of eating, drinking and swallowing and the interplay with breathing, in order to understand what can go wrong as the child develops.

Food and drink are taken into the body through the mouth, into the pharynx and then into the oesophagus. During breathing, air may flow through either the nose or the mouth, through the pharynx, into the larynx and then lungs. The pathways for air and food/fluid cross in the pharynx. The activity of swallowing changes the pharynx from an airway to a food channel. The structures in the mouth, pharynx and larynx have multiple functions in breathing, speaking, biting, chewing and swallowing. The activities of eating, swallowing and breathing need to be tightly coordinated in order to prevent entry of particles of food and/or fluid into the lungs, known as aspiration (Matsuo & Palmer 2008).

Breathing

Respiration continues unnoticed in the background of human activity. The usual rhythms of breathing are interrupted by the activities of eating, drinking and swallowing. The need to swallow food, fluid or saliva will dominate the need to breathe. Breathing briefly stops during swallowing because of the physical closure of the airway and also because of neural suppression of breathing at the brainstem. Different patterns of inhalation and exhalation have been linked to drinking single sips, consecutive swallowing of fluid from a cup and chewing and swallowing food. However, the most typical respiratory pattern in healthy adults is slight inspiration before swallow followed by expiration after the swallow (Martin-Harris 2006). A different pattern is observed in infants such that swallows are equally distributed between the expiratory and inspiratory phases of respiration.

Children with neurodisability may experience difficulties with breathing and respiration. This will influence and interfere with the fine choreography between respiration and eating, drinking and swallowing as well as other areas of function (Kansra & Ugonna 2016; Seddon & Khan 2003). These include:

- Disturbances to the respiratory rhythm affecting the depth of breathing and rhythm over time linked to disturbances to a child's altered neurology

- Obstructions to breathing linked to anatomy or physiology: stertor, stridor, pooling of secretions

- Chronic lung disease of prematurity

- Weak cough and airway clearance because of weak or uncoordinated contraction of expiratory abdominal and intercostal muscles

- Lack of exercise which induces deep breathing which aids clearance of secretions and opens up underventilated lung regions, which leaves the child with neurodisability prone to atelectasis, infection and hypoxaemia

- Respiratory muscle weakness linked to neurodisability and in particular neuromuscular disorders and spinal cord lesions

- Spinal curvature frequently occurs in individuals with all types of neurological disability because of unequal muscle tone and gravity. Chest wall deformity secondary to severe kyphoscoliosis restricts lung function by decreasing chest wall compliance and decreasing the mechanical advantage of the respiratory muscles

Stages of Eating, Drinking and Swallowing

Eating, drinking and swallowing are complex behaviours that involve both volitional and reflexive activities (Matsuo & Palmer 2008). The activity of eating, drinking and swallowing can be divided into different stages according to the location of food or drink as it travels from the mouth, through the throat and into the oesophagus. The activity at each of the different stages does not occur sequentially; there will be overlap between stages in this process. The activity of bringing food and drinking to the mouth will also have an influence on the whole process and needs to be included, particularly in the context of children with neurodisability who are frequently dependent upon assistance from others to eat and drink. This is described in detail in the previous chapter. Disturbances to function at different stages of eating and drinking are outlined in this section.

Anticipatory Stage

The Anticipatory Stage of eating, drinking and swallowing includes emotions, memories, thoughts, actions and intentions that someone brings prior to the stage when food or drink enters the mouth. Personal and environmental factors will influence this stage when external cues from the environment meet an individual's senses (Shune et al. 2016). Disturbances to function at the Anticipatory Stage affect engagement, safety, efficiency and enjoyment of mealtimes.

Awareness, anticipation and motivation

- Altered alertness and awareness affect understanding and response to external cues

- Risk of choking or aspiration linked to reduced awareness

- Efficient rhythms bringing food/drink to mouth may be difficult to establish

- Unmotivated or inefficient self-feeding affects amounts consumed

- Internal experiences of hunger or thirst may not be noticed or present

Readiness to eat/drink

- Experience of fear, pain, upset, anger or lethargy will affect intake

- Aspiration or choking events may occur especially if readiness to eat/drink is overlooked

Sensory information

- Limited or altered sensory information (e.g. vision, hearing, smell, touch) affects anticipatory mouth movements for eating/drinking

- Required movements to accommodate arrival of food, spoon, nipple or teat, or cup at mouth may be disturbed

- Problematic for individuals dependent upon others at mealtimes

- Sensory feedback about physical properties of food/drink in the hand such as size, taste, texture and temperature may not be available to plan and execute requisite movements

- Timing of mouth opening will be affected with impact upon efficiency

- Risk of choking and asphyxiation by individuals with sensory difficulties who eat/drink at speed and in large volumes

Communication

- Limited communication skills affect individuals' ability to make clear requests or regulate mealtime pace

- Limited verbal communication and reduced independence can impact nutritional intake (Fung et al. 2002)

- Ability to express preferences or eat independently may lead to individuals engaging in riskier behaviours with increased risks of choking and aspiration (Chadwick et al. 2006)

Case Study 1 describes difficulties arising for one child at the Anticipatory Stage.

Oral Stage

The Oral Stage includes the processes involved in the mouth to prepare food and drink ready for swallowing (Matsuo & Palmer 2008). Disturbances to function at the Oral Stage affect nutritional intake, as well as efficiency and safety of eating/drinking.

Taking food/fluid into the mouth

- Limited or uncoordinated mouth opening in infancy, difficulties using tongue to secure nipple on palate and initiate downward movement to initiate suction, followed by upward movement to express milk affecting feeding safety and efficiency (Sheppard & Malandraki 2015)

- Limited coordination and range of movement of lips, jaw, facial muscles and tongue affect intake: lips and jaw may remain closed; jaw may clamp down on utensils; tonic bite or tongue thrust may push food/fluid out; challenging to create suction to draw liquid into mouth, or transfer food from front to further into the mouth (Evans Morris & Dunn Klein 2001; Chadwick et al. 2006)

- Limited reflexive suckle swallow movement patterns used to draw food/fluid into mouth, with limited access to volitional movements

Case Study 1: Toby

Diagnosis:

Hypoxic-ischemic encephalopathy and necrotising enterocolitis linked to preterm birth at 28 weeks gestational age. Cerebral palsy diagnosis confirmed age 2 years.

Classification of function at age 7 years:

Gross Motor Function Classification System (GMFCS) IV – Self mobility with limitation (Palisano et al. 1997).

Manual Ability Classification System (MACS) III – Handles objects with difficulty; needs help to prepare and/or modify activities (Eliasson et al. 2006).

Viking Speech Scale II – Speech is imprecise but usually understandable to unfamiliar listener (Pennington et al. 2013).

Communication Function Classification System (CFCS) IV – Inconsistent Sender and/or Receiver with familiar partners (Hidecker et al. 2011).

Eating and drinking ability:

EDACS II – Eats and drinks safely but with some limitations to efficiency (Sellers et al. 2014a).

Toby was spoon fed thin smooth puree with sips of drink between each mouthful because of extreme sensitivity to food smells and sensation of food in his mouth. Environment and carer techniques needed to be consistent in order to encourage Toby to eat and drink without triggering gagging and projectile vomiting, e.g. same relaxing music, no sudden sounds or movements, no strong-smelling food, use of distraction techniques. Toby sometimes liked to feed himself foods such as dry breakfast cereals and bread sticks with his fingers especially when no one expected him to eat.

Toby's extreme sensitivity was addressed with intensive desensitisation programmes by occupational and speech and language therapists over 1 year. This was combined with environmental modifications to reduce carer control and increase Toby's independence at mealtimes with access to finger foods and adapted equipment to feed himself. This led to improved oral intake, elimination of gagging and vomiting at mealtimes, increased participation in mealtimes and greater expressed enjoyment.

Retaining food/fluid in the mouth

- Spillage of food, drink and saliva from lips and into gaps between cheeks and gums (Matsuo & Palmer 2008; Sellers et al. 2014a)

- Food or fluid may prematurely spill over back of tongue into pharynx with increased risk of aspiration (Matsuo & Palmer 2008)

Biting and chewing

- Limited biting of food using precise jaw pressure and lip and tongue movement to transfer food to molars for chewing

- Rhythmical repetitive vertical excursions of jaw in combination with rotary movements of tongue and coordinated activity of lips and cheeks may be challenging (Remijn et al. 2013)

- Limited lateral tongue movement affects movement of food around mouth (Reilly et al. 2000; Matsuo & Palmer 2008; Remijn et al. 2013)

- Individual may bite tongue, cheeks or lips because of limitations in coordinating movements (Matsuo & Palmer 2008)

- Limited ability to alter properties of food and reduce to size suitable for swallowing is linked to choking and asphyxiation

- Hyper-reactive gag reflex may limit intake

- Modification of textures reduces demands at Oral Stage

Initiating the swallow

- Limited elevation of tongue tip behind upper front teeth whilst holding suitably prepared food or fluid on the surface of the tongue will affect ability to initiate swallow

- Limitations to movements required to change area of tongue to palate contact and gradually extend this backwards squeezing food/fluid towards back of the mouth will lead to arhythmical and piecemeal swallowing

- Repeated movements required to clear mouth

- May increase risk of choking and aspiration, and be associated with limited nutritional intake

Case Study 2 describes difficulties arising for one child at the Oral Stage.

Pharyngeal Stage

Whilst the preparatory Oral Stage is primarily volitional, the Pharyngeal Stage is a rapid sequential activity or patterned response taking less than a second to complete (Malandraki et al. 2011a; Matsuo & Palmer 2008). Disturbances to function at the Pharyngeal Stage are particularly linked to safety of eating/drinking although efficiency and enjoyment can also be affected.

Timing of swallow

- Infants with neurodisability may have limitations to suck swallow breathe coordination which includes timing of the swallow (Dodrill & Gosa 2015)

- Limitations may persist with use of limited suckle swallow movement patterns to ingest food/fluid

---

Case Study 2: Mary

Diagnosis:

Worster-Drought syndrome diagnosed age 5 years. Worster-Drought syndrome is a type of cerebral palsy affecting the muscles of the mouth and pharynx leading to difficulties with eating, drinking, swallowing and saliva control, as well as other actions controlled by these muscles.

Classification of function at age 9 years:

GMFCS IV – Walks without limitations.

MACS III – Handles objects easily and successfully.

Viking Speech Scale II – Speech is imprecise but usually understandable to unfamiliar listeners.

CFCS II – Effective but slower paced Sender and Receiver with unfamiliar and familiar partners.

Eating and drinking ability:

EDACS III – Eats and drinks with some limitations to safety; there may be some limitations to efficiency.

Mary was able to efficiently suck and swallow milk from an infant bottle. She relied on bottle feeding for a great deal of her nutritional needs until age 7 years. Her oral movements were restricted to forward/backward tongue movement, no lateral tongue or jaw movement necessary for biting and chewing food and limited lip involvement to retain food/drink in her mouth. After a prolonged weaning period with some choking episodes, she learnt to chew soft lumps and eat soft mashed food. Hard lumps, mixed food textures and fast-flowing thin fluids continued to present choking and aspiration risks to Mary. Food, fluid and saliva loss linked to limited selective lip movement caused Mary some social embarrassment. Mary learnt effective self-management strategies with careful support from family and school staff.

- Altered muscle tone, limited coordination and limited range of movement may delay initiation of swallow (Arvedson 2013; Dodrill & Gosa 2015)

- Repeated attempts at coordinated strong muscle activity may be required to elevate larynx and hyoid bone upward and forward

- May experience particular difficulties swallowing fluids because of delayed pharyngeal swallow initiation (Arvedson 2013)

Clearance of throat

- Muscles in throat may be reduced or asymmetrical where one side of the body is more affected than the other affecting movement of food/fluid through pharynx to upper oesophageal sphincter (Arvedson 2013; Dodrill & Gosa 2015)

- Food and fluid residues may pool in the pharynx before or after swallowing with particular difficulties clearing thick smooth, lumpy or mashed food residues from pharynx with reduced pharyngeal motility (Arvedson 2013)

- Back flow of liquid/food into nasopharynx may occur because of limited or uncoordinated movement of the soft palate (Arvedson 2013)

- Risk that food/fluid residue may enter open airway after swallowing (Arvedson 2013)

Altered pharyngeal and laryngeal sensation

- Disturbances to sensorimotor function in aerodigestive tract will have adverse effects on swallowing safety (Ulualp et al. 2013)

Case Study 3 describes difficulties arising for one child at the Pharyngeal Stage.

Case Study 3: William

Diagnosis:

Degenerative neurological condition of unknown origin following a period of typical development until age 7 years.

Function at age 13 years:

Gradual loss of motor control. At 13 years he was unable to move independently, requiring assistance from others for all transfers. Unable to handle objects. Unable to use speech. Indicated yes/no with distinct eye movements and showed pleasure, pain, sadness, anger with his voice.

Eating and drinking ability:

Gradual loss of function linked to changes throughout William's body with increasing muscle tone, reduced range and coordination of movement in face, mouth, tongue and throat. William gradually reduced the amount he ate and drank; gastrostomy was inserted at 12 years. Aspiration pneumonia and hospitalisation led to recommendation that William no longer eat or drink because of safety concerns. Clinical assessment including use of cervical auscultation supported request for videofluoroscopic swallow study (VFSS). Silent aspiration demonstrated on VFSS when William drank thin fluid because of delays in the pharyngeal stage of swallow and premature entry of fluid into the pharynx. William made repeated attempts to swallow fluid and did not cough to clear fluid from airway. He was able to coordinate oral and pharyngeal stages to manage small volumes of soft-chew food texture, mash and purees. Recommendation was to eat small volumes of food for pleasure and participation in mealtime experiences. Gastrostomy was used to provide all his nutritional and hydrational needs.

Aspiration

Airway protection is critical to swallowing with serious consequences if usual safety mechanisms fail. If the activities of swallowing and breathing are not closely coordinated, it is possible that particles of food/fluid will enter the lungs, known as aspiration (Matsuo & Palmer 2008). The usual protective response to aspiration is a strong reflex coughing or throat clearing. Aspiration may occur if laryngeal sensation is altered or strength of cough and throat clearing is compromised by weak or uncoordinated movement linked to neurodisability (Matsuo & Palmer 2008; Weir et al. 2009). Aspiration events can occur at any of the stages of eating, drinking and swallowing outlined above, including from saliva or gastric refluxate produced in anticipation of food/drink.

It is not possible to observe the sequence of events taking place inside the mouth, throat and larynx when someone eats and drinks. Instrumental measures such as dynamic X-ray (videofluoroscopic swallow studies [VFSS]) and fibreoptic endoscopic evaluation of swallowing (FEES) provide the means to visualise some of these hidden events in a limited time frame. In radiological investigations it is important to distinguish between aspiration, defined as passage of materials through the vocal folds, and laryngeal penetration, defined as passage of materials into the larynx but not through the vocal folds. The term 'silent aspiration' is used when aspiration is visualised using instrumental measures but is not accompanied by coughing, the expected response when food/fluid enters the larynx (Leder et al. 1998; Weir et al. 2009). Aspiration can occur before the swallow linked to early entry of fluids or food into the pharynx or a delay in laryngeal closure after food/fluid has been propelled into the pharynx (Matsuo & Palmer 2008). Aspiration after the swallow may be due to accumulated food and/or fluid residues in the pharynx which are inhaled when breathing resumes.

The consequences of aspiration are highly variable, ranging from no discernible effect through to airway obstruction or severe aspiration pneumonia (Cass et al. 2005; Matsuo & Palmer 2008). Chronic or recurrent respiratory symptoms can arise when there is repeated passage of food/fluid, saliva or gastric refluxate into the lungs (Boesch et al. 2006). A UK-based study examining 'cause of death' as described on the death certificates of people with cerebral palsy found that 22% of deaths resulted from solids or liquids in the lungs or windpipe (Glover & Ayub 2010). Demonstrated aspiration on VFSS or FEES of food or fluid is not always correlated with respiratory morbidity (Cass et al. 2005). Accordingly, it is important to distinguish 'clinically significant' aspiration from a single radiologically demonstrated aspiration or penetration (Arvedson 2013). The diagnosis of chronic pulmonary aspiration is made clinically with some supporting diagnostic evaluations, although the diagnosis may be made after significant lung injury has occurred (Boesch et al. 2006).

Activity

The cultural requirements linked to age expectations can present the child with neurodisability with new challenges. Learning to eat and drink in more upright positions, against the increased pulls of gravity, can cause difficulties (Larnert et al. 1995). A child with neurodisability may be able to safely and efficiently drink from a bottle using well-practised suck swallow breathe synchrony skills; however, prolonged bottle use will clash with what is deemed socially and developmentally appropriate. Drinking fast-flowing liquid from an open cup may be more culturally acceptable but it may increase likelihood of aspiration. Encouragement to develop independent eating and drinking skills may affect the volumes of food and drink consumed and may have an impact on the oral skills that a child with neurodisability can bring to the task.

Participation

It can be challenging for parents of children with neurodisability to cope with their children's altered eating/drinking needs. Where children have limited eating/drinking abilities, their parents can experience difficulties participating in everyday activities (Fung et al. 2002). Individual choice and the wish to participate in usual mealtime experiences may lead to greater levels of risk taking with subsequent compromised health (Chadwick et al. 2006). Professional engagement in problem solving with children with neurodisability and their parents can support fuller participation and reduce conflict.

Chapter 10 outlines the psychosocial aspects of assessment and management.

ASSESSMENT

Techniques for assessing and diagnosing children's eating, drinking and swallowing difficulties associated with neurodisability include clinical evaluation and instrumental investigation. It is important to consider the eating, drinking and swallowing abilities of a child with neurodisability in conjunction with other aspects of function including development, pulmonary health, growth and dietary intake. A multidisciplinary team can provide children and their families with a more comprehensive approach to assessment, treatment and management of eating, drinking and swallowing difficulties.

Clinical Evaluation

Clinical evaluation will include history, physical examination and observation of feeding, eating, drinking and swallowing (Arvedson 2013; Dodrill & Gosa 2015). The use of frameworks and checklists supports clinicians to develop treatment and management plans linked to an understanding of a child's difficulties.

In a recent review of the clinimetrics of feeding measures it was recognised that there was no single measure that represents a systematic and comprehensive evaluation of eating, drinking and swallowing difficulties for the clinical setting (Benfer et al. 2012). As with other areas of function different measurement tools have been developed to measure different aspects of eating and drinking. It is challenging to encapsulate all the different factors outlined here in a single assessment.

See Table 2.1 for details of some standardised clinical assessment tools.

Observation of clinical markers of potential aspiration may be included such as 'wet voice', 'wet breathing' and 'cough' which have been shown to be associated with instrumental observation of oropharyngeal aspiration on thin fluid (Weir et al. 2009). Some clinicians choose to supplement visual evaluation with the use of auditory information from throat sounds (cervical auscultation) to determine when swallowing takes place, as well as changes to sounds, rates and patterns of breathing. Whilst not as accurate as VFSS, it provides additional information not available from observation alone (Frakking et al. 2016). Cervical auscultation can be used to make subtle clinical signs apparent to a wider audience such as parents or carers. It may also be used to support requests for instrumental investigation.

It is a challenge for specialist clinicians to translate the multilayered descriptions of children's eating, drinking and swallowing function into a format that is readily understood by professional colleagues, parents and other stakeholders. Ineffective communication among healthcare professionals has been identified as one of the leading causes of medical errors and patient harm (Dingley et al. 2008). Effective communication is the foundation of any healthcare team. Measurement tools designed to communicate the extent to which children's eating and drinking abilities are limited by neurodisability have been developed but few meet recognised quality standards for health measurement tools (Sellers et al. 2014b). See Dysphagia Disorders Management Scale (DDMS) and Eating and Drinking Ability Classification System (EDACS) in Table 2.2.

The EDACS is an ordinal scale developed to classify usual eating/drinking performance of children with cerebral palsy using key features of safety and efficiency. It follows the design of other popular classification systems describing other areas of function (Palisano et al. 1997; Eliasson et al. 2006; Hidecker et al. 2011; Pennington et al. 2013). It has been developed to be used by parents as well as health professionals, with the potential for clear and consistent information sharing between professionals and parents. There is a significant moderate positive association between children's ability to sit, stand and move measured by the Gross Motor Function Classification System (GMFCS) (Palisano et al. 1997) and their eating and drinking ability measured

Table 2.1 Some standardised clinical assessment tools to measure eating, drinking, feeding and swallowing difficulties

Dysphagia Disorders Survey (DDS) (Sheppard et al. 2014)	• Identify and describe swallowing and feeding disorders • Individuals with developmental disability • Age range 3 years to adulthood • Good clinical utility (Benfer et al. 2012) • Limited reliability data (Benfer et al. 2012) • Users must attend certificated training • Professional use only
Schedule for Oral Motor Assessment (SOMA) (Reilly et al. 2000)	• Standardised procedure for evaluating eating and drinking ability • Enables distinction between young children with or without eating/drinking difficulties • Age range 10–42 months • Lack of sensitivity to certain difficulties linked to neurodisability (Clark et al. 2010) • Not based on usual mealtime performance • Strong psychometric properties (Benfer et al. 2012) • Manualised • Professional use only
Mastication Observation and Evaluation instrument (Remijn et al. 2013)	• Observation and assessment of chewing ability • Children with cerebral palsy • Age range 29–65 months • Content validity and reliability good (Remijn et al. 2013) • Not based on usual mealtime performance • Clinical utility not yet determined • Professional use only
Neonatal Oral Motor Assessment Scale (NOMAS) (Zarem et al. 2013)	• Tool to evaluate neonatal sucking patterns • Age range preterm and term infants • Enables identification of normal, disorganised and dysfunctional oral motor patterns • Substandard reliability with some evidence of construct validity (Zarem et al. 2013) • Users must attend certificated training • Professional use only
Pediatric Eating Assessment Tool (Pedi-EAT) (Thoyre et al. 2014)	• Parent-report measure of problematic eating behaviours • Good content validity with input from researchers, clinicians and parents (Thoyre et al. 2014) • Reliability and other psychometric properties yet to be reported

Table 2.2 Eating and drinking ability severity rating scales

Dysphagia Disorders Management Scale (DDMS) – part of the Dysphagia Disorders Survey (Sheppard et al. 2014)	• 5-level ordinal scale rating severity of disordered feeding and swallowing • Individuals with developmental disability • Based on management needs and health-related outcome • Information from parent questionnaire • Professional use only following certificated training • Limited psychometric properties reported
Eating and Drinking Ability Classification System (EDACS) (Sellers et al. 2014a)	• 5-level ordinal scale to classify eating and drinking ability • Individuals with cerebral palsy • Age range 3 years to adulthood • Based on usual performance at mealtimes • Strong content validity and reliability • For professional and parent use

by EDACS (Sellers et al. 2014a). The association is moderate in that GMFCS level is not sufficient to predict the extent to which someone's eating and drinking ability is affected by cerebral palsy: children who are unable to walk independently may have few limitations to movements required to eat and drink safely and efficiently; some children who are able to walk may experience severe limitations to eating, drinking and swallowing affecting both safety and efficiency.

The lack of agreement about measures of eating and drinking abilities for different populations of children with neurodisability affects estimates of prevalence, likely comorbidities and prediction of future function. Classification systems such as EDACS may be used to stratify and target therapies appropriately for children with similar neurodisabilities (Rosenbaum et al. 2014).

It is possible to describe the oral sensorimotor function of children with neurodisability, but pharyngeal function can only be inferred from a clinical evaluation (Arvedson 2013).

Instrumental Assessment

VFSS and FEES are the most commonly used instrumental measures of swallow function (Dodrill & Gosa 2015). Both assessment techniques provide accurate diagnosis of aspiration and swallowing difficulties in the paediatric population when applied and interpreted by experienced clinicians. Both measures take place within a limited time frame and in unusual environments which can sometimes be challenging for children and their families.

Videofluoroscopy of Swallowing

The VFSS is a radiographic, qualitative, dynamic assessment for assessing the biomechanics of swallowing and the adequacy of airway protection (Sheppard & Malandraki 2015).

Advantages include:

- Food and fluid containing barium can be followed from the mouth into the stomach providing radiographic views of anatomy, physiology, timing, biomechanics and effectiveness of the whole swallow

- Possible to visualise penetration of food/fluid into the larynx above vocal folds and aspiration where material passes through the vocal folds into the trachea

- Child eats and drinks range of food and fluid textures to mimic usual eating and drinking

- VFSS can be used to explore and confirm the effectiveness of selected approaches to intervention such as altered food and fluid consistencies, postural changes and techniques

Limitations include:

- Need for child and parent cooperation in a challenging test environment

- Exposure to ionising radiation

- Limited time frame of the investigation

- Usual eating and drinking is constrained by the need for lateral as well as anterior-posterior fluoroscopic views of the swallow in precise time frames

- Posture support from usual equipment such as metal based head supports may need to be removed or altered in order not to obscure the view of neck

Fibreoptic Endoscopic Evaluations of Swallow

The use of fibreoptic endoscopic evaluations of swallow can take place with sensory testing (FEEST) or without sensory testing (FEES). Investigation using FEES requires the passing of a soft flexible nasal endoscope into the nose and positioning between the soft palate and the epiglottis (Sheppard & Malandraki 2015).

Advantages include:

- Procedure may be tolerable for some children with neurodisability especially if they are used to the regular passing of a nasogastric feeding tube or suction catheter

- Facilitates a view of the oral and pharyngeal anatomy and some swallowing events including for saliva, and usual food and fluid

- Signs of pooling, penetration and aspiration are apparent before or after the swallow

- Sensory stimulation consists of a puff of air delivered to the aryepiglottic folds to test the threshold for laryngeal adductor reflex: sensory thresholds have been shown to be related to presence of aspiration (Ulualp et al. 2013)

- Suitable for children who have never fed orally with concerns about aspiration of saliva, saliva pooling in pharynx or when unable to accept sufficient food for VFSS assessment

- Procedure can be repeated without exposure to ionising radiation

Limitations include:

- Some children may find procedure invasive, upsetting and intolerable

- Need for child and parent cooperation in a challenging test environment

- Limited time frame of the investigation

- Atypical setting for eating and drinking

- During the swallow, pharyngeal contraction obscures the view – moment of 'white out'

DIFFICULTIES, DILEMMAS AND ETHICAL DECISION MAKING

It is essential to think about the whole context of a child's eating and drinking difficulties and the aims of any intervention. A child may have limitations in controlling posture, inefficient movements, limited abilities to chew which may increase risk of choking, and emotional and behavioural associations with eating and drinking. There will also be other important quality of life issues linked to individual choice, parental preference and participation factors.

All of these factors and more are not apparent when swallowing is viewed through an instrumental lens such as videofluoroscopy. Such assessments enable the creation of clear binary distinctions between the presence and absence of aspiration, that is, a swallow that is safe and one that is unsafe, but the results of investigations must be interpreted in the context of the clinical picture. The Royal College of Physicians (2010) challenged health professionals to think more widely about the dilemmas and difficulties associated with limitations to eating, drinking and swallowing – to think about more than just the safety of swallow. Cass et al. (2005) presented a series of case studies examining the pulmonary consequences for children with dysphagia, challenging the assumption that aspiration of food or fluid always leads to respiratory compromise and is always harmful. Aspiration of saliva may also contribute to a compromised respiratory system, even when oral nutrition and hydration is restricted. Furthermore, the contribution of poor oral hygiene to aspiration pneumonia in children who receive enteral nutrition is yet to be explored.

The number one question to consider for multiprofessional teams supporting children with eating and drinking difficulties is 'What are we trying to achieve?' (Royal College of Physicians 2010). The child and their family need to be at the centre of the team's efforts. It may be that oral intake is the main aim of interventions: the child may require modified food or fluid textures, and close attention to be paid to personal and environmental factors, including nutrient-dense food and drink. Tube feeding may be required to supplement or replace oral nutrition and hydration. If someone has an 'unsafe swallow', a risk management approach is required to offer children and their families the best quality of life: this may include the child being offered regular tastes, flavours and smells of food and drink, and good oral care with products that provide choices about smells, flavours and oral sensations. Families will require support and partnership working to minimise the impact on their lives of their child's eating and drinking difficulties, including use of enteral feeding (Craig 2013).

The Four Topic model outlined by Jonsen, Siegler and Winslade in 1982 has been adopted by clinical teams to enhance the clinical and ethical decision making necessary when someone experiences limitations to eating, drinking and swallowing (Sharp & Genesen 1996). Clinical decisions with ethical dilemmas can be enhanced by considering (1) Medical indications, (2) Patient preferences, (3) Contextual factors and (4) Quality of life. Finding a balance between these different factors enables multiprofessional teams, children and their families to work through differences of opinion and potential sources of conflict.

Working in partnership with families of children with neurodisability has been demonstrated to lead to favourable outcomes (Law et al. 2003). Family-centred care is associated with better psychological adjustment; increased parental knowledge about children's development; increased participation by parents in home therapy programmes; increased feelings of competence, self-efficacy and control by parents; increased satisfaction with care provided; and individualised family outcomes. By working in partnership with parents and their children, it will be possible to draw out important social and emotional dimensions of shared mealtime experiences that may not form part of usual medical considerations. Conflicts between parents and healthcare professionals concerning the eating, drinking and swallowing needs of children with neurodisability are not inevitable. Clarity about roles and responsibilities, together with a better understanding of what constitutes risk amid uncertainty, are required in negotiations between health professionals and parents of children with neurodisability (Craig & Higgs 2012).

REFERENCES

Arvedson JC (2013) Feeding children with cerebral palsy and swallowing difficulties. *Eur J Clin Nutr* 67: S9–S12.

Auld ML, Boyd RN, Moseley GL, Ware RS, Johnston LM (2012) Impact of tactile dysfunction on upper-limb motor performance in children with unilateral cerebral palsy. *Arch Phys Med Rehabil* 93(4): 696–702.

Benfer KA, Weir KA, Boyd RN (2012) Clinimetrics of measures of oropharyngeal dysphagia for preschool children with cerebral palsy and neurodevelopmental disabilities: a systematic review. *Dev Med Child Neurol* 54: 784–795.

Boesch RP, Daines C, Willging JP et al. (2006) Advances in the diagnosis and management of chronic pulmonary aspiration in children. *Eur Resp J* 28(4): 847–861.

Cass H, Wallis C, Ryan M, Reilly S, McHugh K (2005) Assessing pulmonary consequences of dysphagia in children with neurological disabilities: when to intervene? *Dev Med Child Neurol* 47(5): 347–352.

Chadwick DD, Jolliffe J, Goldbart J, Burton MH (2006) Barriers to caregiver compliance with eating and drinking recommendations for adults with intellectual disabilities and dysphagia. *J App Res Intellect Dis* 19: 153–162.

Clark M, Harris R, Jolleff N, Price K, Neville BG (2010) Worster-Drought syndrome: poorly recognized despite severe and persistent difficulties with feeding and speech. *Dev Med Child Neurol* 52(1): 27–32.

Craig GM (2013) Psychosocial aspects of feeding children with neurodisability. *Eur J Clin Nutr* 67: S17.

Craig GM, Higgs P (2012) Risk owners & risk managers: dealing with the complexity of feeding children with neurodevelopmental disability. *Health Risk Soc* 14(7): 627–637.

Crary MA (2016) Adult neurologic disorders. In: Groher ME, Crary MA (eds). *Dysphagia: Clinical Management in Adults and Children*, 2nd edn. St Louis, MO: Elsevier Inc, Pt III, Ch 13.

Dingley C, Daugherty K, Derieg MK, Persing R (2008) Improving patient safety through provider communication strategy enhancements. In: Henriksen K, Battles JB, Keyes MA et al. (eds). *Advances in Patient Safety: New Directions and Alternative Approaches (Vol. 3: Performance and Tools)*. Rockville, MD: Agency for Healthcare Research and Quality (US). Available from: https://www.ncbi.nlm.nih.gov/books/NBK43663/.

Dodrill P, McMahon S, Ward E, Weir K, Donovan T, Riddle B (2004) Long-term oral sensitivity and feeding skills of low-risk pre-term infants. *Early Hum Dev* 76(1): 23–37.

Dodrill P, Gosa MM (2015) Pediatric dysphagia: physiology, assessment and management. *Ann Nutr Metab* 66(Suppl. 5): 24–31.

Eliasson AC, Krumlinde-Sundholm L, Rösblad B et al. (2006) The Manual Ability Classification System (MACS) for children with cerebral palsy: scale development and evidence of validity and reliability. *Dev Med Child Neurol* 48: 549–554.

Ertekin C, Keskin A, Kiylioglu N et al. (2001) The effect of head and neck positions on oropharyngeal swallowing: a clinical and electrophysiologic study. *Arch Phy Med Rehab* 82(9): 1255–1260.

Evans Morris S, Dunn Klein M (2001) *Pre-feeding Skills: A Comprehensive Resource for Mealtime Development*, 2nd edn Cambridge, MA: Academic Press.

Frakking TT, Chang AB, O'Grady K, David M, Walker-Smith K, Weir KA (2016) The use of cervical auscultation to predict oropharyngeal aspiration in children: a randomized controlled trial. *Dysphagia* 31: 738–748.

Fung EB, Samson-Fang L, Stallings VA et al. (2002) Feeding dysfunction is associated with poor growth and health status in children with cerebral palsy. *J Am Diet Assoc* 102(3): 361–373.

Gericke T (2006) Postural management for children with cerebral palsy: consensus statement. *Dev Med Child Neurol* 48(4): 244.

Glover G, Ayub M (2010) How people with learning disabilities die. *Improving Health and Lives: Learning Disabilities Observatory.* https://www.researchgate.net/publication/257984926_How_People_With_Learning_Disabilities_Die.

Hidecker MJ, Paneth N, Rosenbaum PL et al. (2011) Developing and validating the Communication Function Classification System for individuals with cerebral palsy. *Dev Med Child Neurol* 53(8): 704–710.

Kansra S, Ugonna K (2016) Fifteen-minute consultation: approach to management of respiratory problems in children with neurodisability. *Arch Dis Child-Ed Pract* 101: 226–231.

Larnert G, Ekberg O (1995) Positioning improves the oral and pharyngeal swallowing function in children with cerebral palsy. *Acta Paediatrica* 84: 689–692.

Law M, Rosenbaum P, King G et al. (2003) How does family-centred service make a difference? https://canchild.ca/system/tenon/assets/attachments/000/001/267/original/FCS3.pdf.

Leder SB, Sasaki CT, Burrell MI (1998) Fiberoptic endoscopic evaluation of dysphagia to identify silent aspiration. *Dysphagia* 13(1): 19–21.

Malandraki GA, Perlman AL, Karampinos DC, Sutton BP (2011a) Reduced somatosensory activations in swallowing with age. *Human Brain Mapping* 32: 730–743.

Malandraki GA, Johnson S, Robbins J (2011b) Functional MRI of swallowing: from neurophysiology to neuroplasticity. *Head & Neck* 33: S14–S20.

Martin-Harris B (2006) Coordination of respiration and swallowing. *GI Motility Online.* https://www.nature.com/gimo/contents/pt1/full/gimo10.html.

Matsuo K, Palmer JB (2008) Anatomy and physiology of feeding and swallowing: normal and abnormal. *Phys Med Rehab Clin North Am* 19(4): 691–707.

Odding E, Roebroeck ME, Stam HJ (2006) Epidemiology of cerebral palsy: incidence,impairments and risk factors. *Dis Rehab* 28(4): 183–191.

Palisano R, Rosenbaum P, Walter S, Russell D, Wood E, Galuppi B (1997) Development and reliability of a system to classify gross motor function in children with cerebral palsy. *Dev Med Child Neurol* 39: 214–223.

Pennington L, Virella D, Mjøen T et al. (2013) Development of The Viking Speech Scale to classify the speech of children with cerebral palsy. *Res Dev Dis* 34(10): 3202–3210.

Ramstad K, Jahnsen R, Skjeldal OH, Diseth TH (2011) Characteristics of recurrent musculoskeletal pain in children with cerebral palsy aged 8 to 18 years. *Dev Med Child Neurol* 53: 1013–1018.

Reilly S, Skuse D, Wolke D (2000) *SOMA: Schedule for Oral Motor Assessment*. London: Whurr Publishers Ltd.

Remijn L, Speyer R, Groen BE, Holtus PC, van Limbeek J, Nijhuis-van der Sanden MW (2013) Assessment of mastication in healthy children and children with cerebral palsy: a validity and consistency study. *J Oral Rehab* 40: 336–347.

Rommel N, De Meyer AM, Feenstra L, Veereman-Wauters G (2003) The complexity of feeding problems in 700 infants and young children presenting to a tertiary care institution. *J Pediatr Gastroent Nutr* 37(1): 75–84.

Rosenbaum P, Paneth N, Leviton A et al. (2007). A report: the definition and classification of cerebral palsy April 2006. *Dev Med Child Neurol* S109: 8–14.

Rosenbaum P, Eliasson AC, Hidecker MJ, Palisano RJ (2014) Classification in childhood disability: focusing on function in the 21st century. *J Child Neurol* 29(8): 1036–1045.

Royal College of Physicians (2010). *Oral Feeding Difficulties and Dilemmas: A Guide to Practical Care, Particularly Towards the End of Life*. https://www.rcplondon.ac.uk/projects/outputs/oral-feeding-difficulties-and-dilemmas.

Seddon PC, Khan Y (2003) Respiratory problems in children with neurological impairment. *Arch Dis Child* 88: 75–78.

Sellers D, Mandy A, Pennington L, Hankins M, Morris C (2014a). Development and reliability of system to classify the eating and drinking ability of people with cerebral palsy. *Dev Med Child Neurol* 56: 245–251.

Sellers D, Pennington L, Mandy A, Morris C (2014b) A systematic review of ordinal scales used to classify the eating and drinking abilities of individuals with cerebral palsy. *Dev Med Child Neurol* 56: 313–322.

Sharp HM, Genesen LB (1996) Ethical decision-making in dysphagia management. *Am J Speech-Lang Path* 5: 15–22.

Sheppard JJ, Hochman R, Baer C (2014) The dysphagia disorder survey: validation of an assessment for swallowing and feeding function in developmental disability. *Res Dev Dis* 35(5): 929–942.

Sheppard JJ, Malandraki GA (2015) Pediatric dysphagia. In: Mankekar G (ed.). *Swallowing – Physiology, Disorders, Diagnosis and Therapy*. New Delhi: Springer Inc., pp. 161–188.

Shune SE, Moon JB, Goodman SS (2016) The effects of age and preoral sensorimotor cues on anticipatory mouth movement during swallowing. *J Speech Lang Hearing Res* 59(2): 195–205.

Spence C (2015) Eating with our ears: assessing the importance of sounds of consumption on our perception and enjoyment of multisensory flavour experiences. *Flavour* 4(3). https://flavourjournal.biomedcentral.com/articles/10.1186/2044-7248-4-3.

Sullivan PB, Juszczak E, Lambert BR, Rose M, Ford-Adams ME, Johnson A (2002) Impact of feeding problems on nutritional intake and growth: Oxford Feeding Study II. *Dev Med Child Neurol* 44(7): 461–467.

Thoyre SM, Pados BF, Park J et al. (2014) Development and content validation of the Pediatric Eating Assessment Tool (Pedi-EAT). *Am J Speech-Lang Path* 23: 46–59.

Ulualp S, Brown A, Sanghavi R, Rivera-Sanchez Y (2013) Assessment of laryngopharyngeal sensation in children with dysphagia. *Laryngoscope* 123(9): 2291–2295.

Weir K, McMahon S, Barry L, Masters IB, Chang AB (2009) Clinical signs and symptoms of oropharyngeal aspiration and dysphagia in children. *Eur Resp J* 33(1): 604–611.

Weir KA, Bell KL, Caristo F et al. (2013) Reported eating ability of young children with cerebral palsy: is there an association with gross motor function? *Arch Phys Med Rehabil* 94(3): 495–502.

World Health Organization (2001) *International Classification of Functioning, Disability and Health.* Geneva: World Health Organization.

Zafeiriou DI (2004) Primitive reflexes and postural reactions in the neurodevelopmental examination. *Pediatr Neurol* 31(1): 1–8.

Zarem C, Kidokoro H, Neil J, Wallendorf M, Inder T, Pineda R (2013) Psychometrics of the neonatal oral motor assessment scale. *Dev Med Child Neurol* 55(12): 1115–1120.

CHAPTER 3

Oral Health and Sialorrhea

Amy Hughes, Isabelle Chase and Laurie Glader

INTRODUCTION

Children with neurodevelopmental disabilities, particularly those with neuromuscular disorders such as cerebral palsy (CP) or myopathies, frequently have challenges associated with oral health and difficulty managing their secretions. This chapter seeks to outline the scope of these challenges, highlighting practical aspects of assessment and intervention for the general practitioner who may provide care for this population of children.

ORAL HEALTH

There are no intraoral anomalies unique to children with neurodevelopmental disorders; however, there are several conditions related to oral health that have been found to be more common than in the general population. When present, they are often severe and may contribute to sialorrhea and difficulties with feeding. Establishment of a dental home by the child's first birthday is recommended to ensure the child with neurodevelopmental conditions receives comprehensive oral health care, including prevention of dental disease and timely trauma care. The American Academy of Pediatrics has produced a clinical report on oral health in children with disabilities which provides practical guidelines for care (Norwood et al. 2013).

Dental Caries

Although there is a paucity of well-controlled studies and the data regarding dental caries in primary teeth is conflicting, the data for permanent teeth suggests that children with neurodevelopmental disorders have a higher rate of dental caries (Botti Rodrigues dos Santos et al. 2003). Food consistency, frequent intake of fermentable carbohydrates, difficulty with chewing and swallowing, food pouching, ingestion of sugar-laden liquid medications and inadequate oral hygiene have been shown to contribute to poor dental health in patients with neurodevelopmental disabilities. Dental caries may lead to pain, infection, tooth loss and a subsequent alteration in the ability to chew hard foods (Chauncey et al. 1984). Drooling may increase as it becomes more painful to close the teeth.

Malocclusion

Children with neurodevelopmental disorders have at least twice the risk of a malocclusion compared to the general population (Franklin et al. 1996). This may exacerbate sialorrhea and impact feeding and swallowing. Excessive overjet (protrusion of the maxillary incisors, Fig. 3.1a), anterior open bite, constriction of the palate leading to a posterior crossbite and a class II malocclusion have been observed most frequently. Development and severity of malocclusion is often multifactorial. Open mouth posture, chronic mouth breathing (Souki et al. 2009), tongue thrust, poor oromotor function,

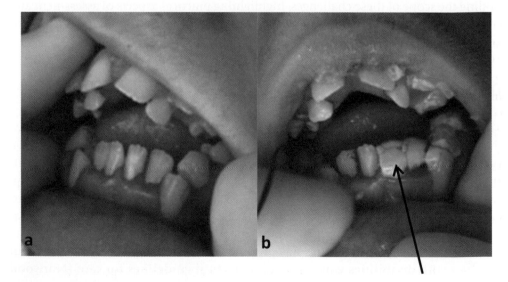

Figure 3.1 Dental images from a patient with cerebral palsy. a: Increased overjet and open bite. b: Dental calculus (arrow) and bleeding.

habitual lip incompetence (Miamoto et al. 2010) and head position (Martinez-Mihi et al. 2014) have all been implicated. With age the malocclusion tends to worsen and as the palate becomes more constricted it prevents the tongue from making proper contact with the anterior hard palate, which is necessary for one of the first phases in swallowing.

The literature is scant with regard to orthodontic treatment in children with neurodevelopmental disabilities and is limited to case reports. For any child potentially undergoing orthodontic treatment, there are some basic issues to consider. This includes need for treatment (aesthetic versus functional), optimal oral hygiene and dental health, parent/guardian commitment and the child's ability to tolerate care. Risk of relapse must also be taken into account prior to initiating treatment. The relapse rate for anterior open bite correction may be as high as 30% and can be complicated by an atypical swallowing pattern and mouth breathing (Wriedt et al. 2009). Although orthodontic treatment is feasible in children with neurodevelopmental disabilities, careful patient selection is imperative as success will not only depend on the basic requirements noted above, but also on the underlying neuromuscular dysfunction, abnormal swallowing pattern (tongue thrust) and persistent mouth breathing.

Oral Hygiene and Periodontal Health

A systematic review of the literature (Diéguez-Pérez et al. 2016) indicates that the oral hygiene (presence of plaque, calculus and food debris) in children with CP is worse than healthy controls (Fig. 3.1b); however, there is conflicting evidence regarding gingival health (gingival inflammation, erythema and bleeding). Gingival hyperplasia and associated bleeding occurs more frequently with the use of antiepileptic medications, but are exacerbated by poor oral hygiene and accumulation of dental calculus (Addy et al. 1983). Children with neurodevelopmental disorders typically depend on their caregivers to care for their teeth. Uncontrolled head movements, gagging, persistent biting reflex, inability to spit, gastroesophageal reflux and brusher fear of causing aspiration may all contribute to inadequate brushing and flossing which, in turn, exacerbates plaque and calculus accumulation.

Hegde et al. (2008) also found that the severity of drooling may impact gingival health. Children with CP and drooling had significantly more calculus than children with CP who did not drool. In children with severe calculus accumulation, poor hydration may be a contributing factor (Botti Rodrigues dos Santos et al. 2011).

Children who are fed either partially or totally by gastronomy tube (GT) have more calculus than children who are able to tolerate oral feeding, despite acceptable oral hygiene practices. *H influenza* has been shown to be significantly higher in patients fed by GT and the presence of calculus is significantly related to aspiration pneumonia (Jawadi et al. 2004). Thus, calculus may place children with neurodevelopmental disorders at a significant systemic health risk. Careful removal in the clinical setting with dental scalers on a frequent basis is recommended. For severe calculus, removal may be necessary in the operating room so that the airway can be properly protected.

Erosion

It is important to rule out gastroesophageal reflux disease (GERD) as a cause of sialorrhea, as uncontrolled GERD leads to displacement of saliva from the tooth and a reduction in the pH of the oral cavity. Loss of the protective coating of the saliva at the tooth surface along with a decreased pH, over time, leads to dissolution of the minerals at the tooth surface and, ultimately, dental erosion. This surface damage is largely irreversible (Ranjitkar et al. 2012), and in combination with bruxism can lead to significant tooth wear, an increased risk for dental caries, pain and sensitivity to both thermal (cold/hot foods) and chemical (sugar) stimuli. Although the long-term effects on the oral mucosa are unknown, chronic, uncontrolled GERD can lead to epithelia atrophy of the oral mucosa.

Bruxism

A systematic review (Diéguez-Pérez et al. 2016) indicates that children with CP present with bruxism (parafunctional tooth grinding or clenching) significantly more than the general population. Bruxism can lead to tooth wear, fractured teeth, joint pain, muscle pain, fatigue and headaches. Bruxism may be related to anticonvulsant medication use, particularly with barbiturates – for example, phenobarbital (Ortega et al. 2014). Bruxism in combination with erosion from gastroesophageal reflux can be detrimental to the dentition. A systematic review shows there is insufficient evidence to support pharmacotherapy to reduce bruxism that occurs during sleep (Macedo et al. 2014). Additionally, there is insufficient evidence that occlusal splints reduce bruxism during sleep (Macedo et al. 2007); however, splints may protect the teeth from abnormal or excessive wear (attrition). Although occlusal splints or mouth guards do not stop bruxism, they can provide protection to the teeth. However, for the patient with dysphagia or gagging, the extra bulk of these appliances may make them uncomfortable or unwearable. There is limited literature related to the use of botulinum toxin in the management of bruxism. Case reports of neuromuscular blocking of the masseter and temporalis muscles with botulinum toxin have shown success in reducing bruxism activity in patients with CP (Manzano et al. 2004).

Trauma

Children with neurodevelopmental disorders are more susceptible to dental trauma, particularly to the maxillary anterior teeth, due to the increased overjet and inadequate lip coverage of these teeth (Corrêa-Faria et al. 2016). Poor motor coordination with falls and loss of stability during transfer from the wheelchair are associated with a higher incidence of dental trauma (Botti Rodrigues dos Santos & Souza 2009). Trauma may result in displacement of the teeth, pain, infection and tooth loss, and the inability to chew. Depending on the dental injury, time plays a critical role in treatment success. Teeth that have been avulsed should be re-implanted immediately, ideally at the scene of the accident, and no greater than one hour after the trauma, followed by placement of a dental splint for 2–4 weeks. When teeth cannot be re-implanted at the scene of the trauma, they should be transported in a medium that helps to preserve the periodontal ligament cells which are necessary for reattachment of the tooth within the alveolar bone. Cold milk is biocompatible with the periodontal ligament cells, thus caregivers should be instructed to place the tooth in cold milk and present to their dentist immediately. Root canal therapy will be required within 7–10 days.

Teeth that are displaced but not avulsed are similarly dependent on time for success. When a tooth is displaced it needs to be repositioned and splinted for 2–4 weeks. Delaying care reduces the ability of the dentist to reposition the tooth to its proper position.

Fractured teeth are less time dependent with regards to intervention and can be successfully treated up to 48 hours after the injury. However, if the fracture has exposed the nerve/pulp of the tooth, this may cause significant pain and care should not be delayed if at all possible.

SIALORRHEA

Background and Assessment

While data on the prevalence of sialorrhea is not available for the diverse and broad population of children with neurodevelopmental disabilities, it has been perhaps best studied in children with CP. In this population, drooling varies depending on severity of motor function and ranges from 10% to 58% (Dias et al. 2016). Table 3.1 details the assessment of patients with sialorrhea. In patients with CP, drooling typically occurs secondary to poor oromotor control in the setting of bulbar and facial muscle dysfunction resulting in abnormal swallowing control, reduced swallowing frequency, altered intraoral sensation and difficulty with lip closure. In rare cases, saliva may be overproduced such as in the presence of active dental concerns (abscesses, caries), gastroesophageal reflux disease, certain antiepileptic medications or frequent mouthing of objects. The degree of sialorrhea can vary, depending on fatigue, positioning, hunger, thirst or emotional state.

Sialorrhea technically refers to increased saliva in the mouth, and may be divided into anterior and posterior manifestations. Drooling is a term typically used to denote anterior

Table 3.1 Assessment of sialorrhea in patients with neurodevelopmental disorders

Component of assessment	Details	Implications
History	Medications (especially benzodiazepines); respiratory symptoms including chronic cough, noisy breathing, need for suctioning, history of respiratory infections; evidence of gastroesophageal reflux disease; craniofacial differences; oral health concerns; environmental allergies	Potential opportunity to: (1) identify risk factors (2) identify posterior drooling (3) intervene with triggers
Motor ability	Posture and head control, swallowing coordination (including ability to swallow on demand), lip closure	Identification of possible factors possibly contributing to sialorrhea which might be treatable (enhanced positioning, lip closure skills)
Quantification of sialorrhea	Number of bibs, frequency of chin wiping, Teacher Drooling Scale score	Important for gauging impact of intervention over time
Identification of type of sialorrhea	Anterior vs posterior, based on history and physical	Critical to determining treatment direction
Self-efficacy	Cognitive ability, motivation, ability to wipe mouth independently	Potential opportunity for behavioural or oromotor therapeutic interventions

sialorrhea, and relates to the unintentional loss of saliva from the mouth. Many typically developing children drool until age 2 and even a bit beyond; abnormal drooling generally suggests drooling beyond age 4. Anterior drooling can have a variety of challenging repercussions but is generally not jeopardising to a child's medical stability. In contrast, posterior drooling may not be visible, making it more difficult to diagnose, but may have serious physiological sequelae. It is prudent for the clinician caring for children with neurodevelopmental disabilities to be aware of the different manifestations of sialorrhea and its management.

Anterior drooling by definition is visible. It can be quantified in a variety of ways utilising established metrics. Most of these scales are utilised in research and may not be practical for office use, but one subjective scale which the authors find particularly useful clinically is the Teacher Drooling Scale (TDS) first published by Camp-Bruno et al. in 1989. The TDS ranks the degree of anterior sialorrhea on a 5-point scale, 1 being completely dry and 5 demonstrating continuous spillage of saliva. In lieu of using a formal scale, anterior drooling severity can be assessed by quantifying the number of clothing or bib changes a child needs over the course of the day. The significance of quantifying anterior drooling lies in establishing a baseline for comparison if an intervention is to be implemented.

Anterior drooling has a number of potential medical and social implications. Medical side effects include skin breakdown or chafing and candida infections. It can also be malodorous. From a social perspective, excessive anterior drooling may interfere with schoolwork or the use of technology and other items that might be placed in front of the child. Importantly, but sometimes overlooked, anterior drooling can have a tremendous impact on a child's social relationships and self-esteem. At times, the impact extends beyond the child to other family members who may experience exhaustion from constant reminders to the child to wipe his or her chin, frequent assistance with this task, doing excessive laundry, and who may bear the burden of being aware of the psychosocial impact of drooling on their child. Any of these sequelae merit consideration of treatment.

Posterior drooling, in contrast to anterior drooling, is not visible and can be more challenging to diagnose. While it may accompany anterior drooling, this is not always the case. Many children with neurodevelopmental disabilities have poor nuchal strength and, depending on the positioning of their head, saliva may flow anteriorly and out of the mouth or posteriorly, oftentimes pooling in the oropharynx and hypopharynx. The child with dysphagia may not only have difficulty swallowing his or her secretions, resulting in pooling, but may be at increased risk for aspiration.

Diagnosis of posterior drooling relies heavily on history, clinical impression and physical exam. A history of frequent coughing, gagging, choking, chest congestion or 'gurgling' sounds reported by caregivers should raise concern for the possibility of posterior drooling. The child who has anterior drooling during the day but none at night may in fact be pooling when his or her position is changed. Additional history of recurrent respiratory infections, persistent cough, or asthma symptoms should raise suspicion for aspiration. On routine examination it may be evident that there is copious saliva in the posterior oropharynx. True identification of aspiration risk is less obvious, however. An otolaryngologist has more sophisticated capability for examining the oromotor structure and may potentially be able to identify aspiration of secretions by fibreoptic nasopharyngoscopy and laryngoscopy. Rarely, a radionuclide salivagram in which tracer is deposited into the mouth and tracked may be useful for formally documenting aspiration of secretions. Imaging obtained an hour after tracer is introduced may reveal that it has, in fact, entered the bronchial tree, supporting a diagnosis of aspiration. Usually such formal documentation is not necessary and the clinician can develop adequate suspicion on the basis of history and physical presentation alone to determine whether or not to intervene.

Potential treatable reasons for sialorrhea should be ruled out, such as poorly controlled gastroesophageal reflux disease, medication side effect or an inadequate seating system. As such, evaluation by a number of providers with differing expertise can provide the most robust approach to diagnosis and management. A paediatrician can obtain a thorough history, evaluate basic neurological control and/or deficits, and pay particular notice to respiratory and gastrointestinal concerns. A speech pathologist has expertise to evaluate lip closure and swallowing coordination and may also look at posture, while a dentist can rule out possible triggering issues, such as an abscess, extensive caries or malocclusion. An otolaryngologist can be helpful in identifying nasal obstruction as a contributor to open mouth posture in addition to potentially observing aspiration directly, as outlined above. Some teams include a psychologist to assess impact of sialorrhea on the child and family as well as readiness for specific interventions.

Once comorbidities potentially contributing to a child's sialorrhea are identified treatment should be initiated. If sialorrhea persists despite treatment, direct management of the sialorrhea itself should be considered, including pharmacological and more invasive interventions such as botulinum toxin injections or surgery. The American Academy of Cerebral Palsy and Developmental Medicine has a care pathway devoted to the evaluation and treatment of sialorrhea which can be found at https://www.aacpdm.org/publications/care-pathways/sialorrhea.

Management

Multiple interventions have been described for the management of sialorrhea. To manage anterior drooling, providers may begin by considering behavioural therapy, oral motor therapy and oral appliances. Typically, these interventions are most effective in patients who are cognitively able to participate in therapy. Additional management options for anterior or posterior drooling, or for individuals with a combination of both, include pharmacological interventions, botulinum toxin injections and surgical procedures. Because of a lack of well-powered and well-designed studies examining these interventions, there has been no clear consensus on which treatments are the safest and most effective. The best existing evidence examines the roles of pharmacological interventions and botulinum toxin injections. What follows is an overview of available interventions, from least to more invasive.

Therapeutic Interventions and Oral Appliances

The goal of behavioural therapy is to alter the frequency or type of a specific behaviour. For drooling, therapy specifically targets swallowing frequency and wiping of the chin and mouth area. Instructions, prompts and cues are set up to make patients aware of the target behaviour; positive feedback, automatic reinforcement and negative reinforcement are used following the target behaviour to reinforce control (Van der Burg et al. 2007). For behavioural therapy to be effective, caregivers should apply techniques daily as intermittent reinforcement has no lasting effect (Van der Burg 2007). For patients and families with positive attitudes as well as a favourable social setting for continuous reinforcement, behavioural therapy may be an effective strategy.

For children who are motivated and able to follow directions, oral motor therapy may be helpful. It focuses on increasing individual awareness, strength and coordination of the oromotor mechanism (Sjogreen et al. 2018). This approach uses active exercises (strength training, active range of motion, stretching), passive exercises (massage, stroking and sensory stimulation such as tapping, application of heat or cold and vibration) (Arvedson et al. 2010). While there are no reported side effects, there is limited evidence supporting its use. Prior to starting therapy, providers need to address abnormalities with patient posture and positioning as well as medical comorbidities such as occlusion abnormalities, medication side effects, and nasal/oropharyngeal obstruction.

Oral appliances for the management of drooling may be used in patients over the age of 6 years to help improve oral motor function. There is no consensus on the type of appliance and necessary duration of treatment, and poor compliance is common. Overall, the literature supporting the use of oral appliances is limited to lower levels of evidence including case studies and retrospective reviews.

Pharmacological Interventions

Medication is often the first intervention used to manage drooling. The majority of pharmacological interventions prescribed are anticholinergic medications which decrease saliva production by inhibiting the salivary glands. Commonly used medications include glycopyrronium bromide, hyoscine hydrobromide patches, trihexyphenidyl hydrochloride, atropine sulfate and benztropine. Use of inhaled ipratropium bromide is favoured by some clinicians; however, there is currently no available efficacy data to support its use in the management of drooling. Glycopyrronium bromide and hyoscine hydrobromide patches are the most frequently used and studied medications. There are limitations in the literature supporting most of these agents and all but glycopyrronium bromide are used in an off-label manner.

A randomised, placebo-controlled Phase III clinical trial examining the efficacy of glycopyrronium bromide solution performed in 2012 (Zeller et al. 2012) showed that patients taking glycopyrronium bromide had a significantly higher response rate than those patients in the placebo group. Most frequently reported side effects included dry mouth, constipation and vomiting. Additional prospective studies have supported this improvement in sialorrhea, but have also shown a dose dependent increase in adverse events, with 20% of children stopping the medication because of behavioural problems, constipation, xerostomia or urinary retention (Mier et al. 2000).

Controlled clinical trials examining the efficacy of hyoscine hydrobromide in decreasing drooling have also been performed (Jongerius et al. 2004). While effective, concerns

Table 3.2 Dosing and complications of pharmacological interventions for sialorrhea

Medication	Dose	Complications
Glycopyrronium bromide	0.02–0.1mg/kg TID[a] (commercially available as 1mg/5ml) Consider titration 0.02mg/kg/dose increase by 0.02mg/kg/dose weekly until effect or max dose of 0.1mg/kg/dose not to exceed 3 mg/dose	• Dry mouth (18–40%) • Constipation (18–30%) • Vomiting (30%) • Nasal obstruction (30%) • Behaviour changes (23%) • Urinary retention (13%)
Hyoscine hydrobromide[b]	Transdermal Patch (1mg–1.5mg depending on formulation/3-day administration)	• Xerostomia (66.7%) • Restlessness (35.6%) • Somnolence (35.6%) • Blurred vision (20%) • Confusion (20%)
Sublingual atropine eyedrops[b]	Atropine ophthalmic 0.5% 1 drop (0.25mg) sublingually up to TID (for patients 10–19kg) 2 drops sublingually up to TID (for patients > or = 20kg) (Dias 2017)	• Difficult administration • Xerostomia • Behaviour changes

[a]TID = three times daily
[b]Off label use

regarding adverse events are greater with use of hyoscine hydrobromide than with glycopyrronium bromide (Parr et al. 2014). Because of its delivery using a patch system, titration is challenging. There is emerging evidence that glycopyrronium bromide is better tolerated than hyoscine hydrobromide (Parr et al. 2018).

Sublingual administration of atropine ophthalmic drops is also often considered as a medical management option. A prospective study examining the effect of the medication on drooling was performed in children with a variety of disabilities (Norderyd et al. 2017). The authors noted a decrease in unstimulated salivary secretion rates from baseline. Side effects included xerostomia and behaviour changes. There were no irreversible side effects, but caregivers complained of administration difficulty. A recent non-placebo-controlled open trial further supported atropine as an effective intervention to treat sialorrhea in children and adolescents with CP (Dias et al. 2017). Further study in a randomised control manner is indicated. Please see Table 3.2 for dosing guidelines.

Botulinum Toxin Injections

Botulinum toxin injections given in a localised manner denervate the salivary glands and have the benefit of no systemic anticholinergic effects. In children this is often performed using ultrasound guidance under general or local anaesthesia. An effect may be seen within 72 hours, with the maximum effect typically seen between 2–8 weeks. Improvement typically lasts between 4–6 months. There is no unified protocol for dosing; however, a recently published study recommended injecting 15U/gland in patients <15kg, 20U/gland for patients weighing 15–25kg and 25U/gland for a weight >25kg (Lungrenet al. 2016). Repeat injections are typically necessary for long-term saliva control.

Several controlled and uncontrolled trials have been published on the use of botulinum toxin for the management of sialorrhea (Jongerius et al. 2004; Khan et al. 2011). Authors have described submandibular gland injections or parotid gland injections alone, as well as combined four-gland injections. Efficacy rates for parotid gland injections or submandibular gland injections alone range between 50–55% (Bothwell et al. 2002; Scheffer et al. 2010). When submandibular and parotid gland injections are performed in combination an improved response has been demonstrated. Most commonly reported side effects include thickened saliva and difficulty swallowing (Reid et al. 2008).

Although the available literature supports the use of botulinum toxin injections for management of sialorrhea, the studies lack homogeneity and there continues to be no unified protocol.

Surgical Interventions

In patients with profuse, consistent anterior drooling despite conservative treatment and patients with persistent posterior drooling with either a history or high risk of developing chronic lung disease, surgical interventions should be considered. Goals of surgical management include redirecting salivary flow through rerouting or eliminating salivary flow through either ligation of salivary ducts or excision of salivary glands.

The most commonly performed procedures include duct ligation, submandibular duct (SMD) rerouting +/- sublingual gland (SLG) excision, and submandibular gland excision (SMGE) +/- parotid duct ligation (PDL). Posterior drooling is a contraindication for SMD rerouting since the procedure results in further accumulation of secretions in the posterior pharynx in a child at risk of aspiration. Potential complications include sialadenitis (salivary gland infection) following duct ligation, lingual nerve injury or ranula (blocked sublingual gland) formation with SMD rerouting +/- SLG excision and lingual or marginal mandibular nerve injury during SMG excision.

Only retrospective reviews of surgical interventions have been performed. Data reviewing two, three or four-duct ligations have demonstrated variable outcomes (Reedet al. 2009) with the largest concern being recurrence. One review estimated recurrence to be as high as 68% (Martin & Conley 2007). Outcomes following SMGE performed alone or in combination with PDL have been better. A meta-analysis by Reed et al. evaluating all surgical treatments of sialorrhea found a generally high success rate following SMGE alone (62–66%) as well as in combination with PDL (75–100%) (Reed et al. 2009). Success rates of SMD rerouting +/– SLG excision are similar to those reported with SMGE (Reed et al. 2009).

In general, reported caregiver satisfaction has been highest for patients after SMD rerouting with SLG excision or SMGE with PDL and lowest following duct ligation procedures. Postoperative anticholinergic use has also been highest following four-duct ligation, likely secondary to the recurrence rate (Stamataki et al. 2008). For individuals who have failed the above-mentioned surgical interventions who continue to experience salivary aspiration and complications related to this such as chronic lung disease, caregivers may consider tracheotomy or, in severe refractory cases, laryngotracheal separation.

Each of these surgical techniques may be associated with potential risks and caregivers must be counselled thoroughly regarding realistic expectations of outcomes. However, salivary gland surgery often presents a reasonable treatment option for patients who have not been responsive for one reason or another to less invasive interventions.

SUMMARY

Children with neurodevelopmental conditions are at risk for a wide variety of oral health concerns which can impact feeding and management of secretions. Additionally, they may have sialorrhea for primary reasons related to oromotor dysfunction. There are significant psychosocial and medical consequences of sialorrhea. Being familiar with the presentation, assessment and treatment options for this important clinical entity benefits all practitioners who care for children with neurodevelopmental conditions.

Note: The authors wish to acknowledge the work of the entire international team who created the sialorrhea care pathway supported through the AACPDM which provided an invaluable foundation for elements of this chapter.

Key Points

1. Children with neurodevelopmental conditions have an increased risk for oral health problems including dental caries, malocclusion, gingival hyperplasia, erosion, bruxism and trauma. These conditions may contribute to sialorrhea and difficulties with feeding.

2. Establishment of a dental home by the child's first birthday is recommended to ensure the child with neurodevelopmental conditions receives comprehensive oral health care, including prevention of dental disease and timely trauma care.

3. Sialorrhea is common in children with neurodevelopmental disabilities and has been documented in 10–58% of children with CP. Initial assessment should rule out treatable triggers such as dental caries or GERD prior to pursuing longitudinal management with the available interventions.

4. Posterior drooling is associated with more clinically significant morbidity, is more challenging to assess than anterior drooling and is often diagnosed by history and exam without additional studies.

5. Anticholinergic medications are the most commonly prescribed medications for drooling management, with recent studies suggesting that glycopyrronium bromide has a better side effect profile than hyoscine hydrobromide and should be considered first line.

6. Botulinum toxin injections to the salivary glands take effect within the first 72 hours, with maximum effect between 2–8 weeks and an average length of improvement of 22 weeks. Reported efficacy is between 68–80% for four-gland injections.

7. Surgical intervention should be considered in patients with consistent profuse anterior drooling refractory to more conservative treatment options or posterior drooling with concerns for chronic lung disease. Evidence suggests that submandibular duct rerouting with sublingual gland excision and submandibular gland excision with or without parotid duct ligation are more effective than duct ligation alone.

Case Study 1: Sam

Sam is a complex non-verbal 15-year-old male with spastic quadriplegia, intellectual disability, gastroesophageal reflux, constipation and recurrent aspiration pneumonia. He has had a fundoplication. Sam eats pureed foods two to three times per day but essentially all nutrition and hydration are administered via a GT. He presents for a dental examination on referral from his primary care physician. His parents have avoided taking him to the dentist for the last few years because their previous dentist was unable to examine him easily and was not accustomed to treating children with special healthcare needs. They were also finding it increasingly difficult to transfer him out of his wheelchair into the dental chair.

Parental concerns are the following:

1. *The appearance of the teeth. Mother feels that despite brushing, his teeth appear 'yellow' and there is a build-up on the teeth.*
2. *Brushing is extremely difficult because he bites down on the toothbrush and he 'gags a lot.' They also see a lot of blood with brushing.*
3. *When they are able to brush, they do not use toothpaste because 'he can't spit' and they are worried he will aspirate.*

Sam was examined in his wheelchair with the chair semi-reclined to avoid any unnecessary transfers. His parents helped to gently hold the hands during the exam. He was noted to have severe yellow dental calculus covering the crowns of most of his teeth. His gingival tissues were inflamed and friable and bled easily with tooth brushing. There were no dental caries and no other pathology noted.

Recommendations:

1. *Removal of the dental calculus. This can be accomplished in the dental clinic typically, but given the severity due to many years of no dental cleanings, the dentist recommended removing the calculus in the operating room under general anaesthesia to allow for airway protection.*

2. *To prevent recurrence of the calculus, dental recalls for professional cleanings were recommended every 3 months, coupled with adequate home care.*

3. *Bleeding of the gingiva occurs when the gingiva are inflamed (gingivitis). This increases with calculus and plaque accumulation. Removing the calculus followed by daily plaque control with brushing should reduce or eliminate the appearance of bleeding. Chlorhexidine gluconate 0.12% may be used 2x/day, for a period of 10–14 days when there is significant gingival bleeding. The use of chlorhexidine will also help to reduce plaque and calculus formation. If it is to be used long term, it should be used for 2 weeks on/2 weeks off to reduce the risk of staining. If staining does occur it is reversible with a professional dental cleaning. These recommendations were given to the family.*

4. *At home, parents were told they could use a small smear of tartar control, fluoride-containing toothpaste. Tartar control toothpastes are ones that contain sodium pyrophosphate and help to reduce the formation of calculus. There is no need to spit out or rinse after brushing. Leaving a film of toothpaste on the teeth will be more beneficial in preventing cavities.*

5. *To prevent biting down on the brush, parents were told to choose times when Sam is most relaxed and having less involuntary movements. This may be outside the conventional times for brushing, but should help with reducing anxiety. Additionally, a mouth prop may be used to help prevent biting down. Soft mouth props may be purchased (e.g. Open Wide® disposable mouth prop) or the parents can fabricate one by stacking five or six tongue depressors together and wrapping at one end with medical tape to provide a soft surface.*

6. *Many parents are concerned with 'gagging' during brushing, like Sam's parents. If regurgitation is happening, ensure the mouth is being suctioned while brushing. For some patients, placing a few grains of salt on the tip of the tongue encourages swallowing. This can be repeated during the brushing process. Suction toothbrush systems that can be attached directly to a home suction system are also available for purchase from medical supply companies.*

Case Study 2: Nathan

Nathan is a 5-year-old male with a history of a chromosomal deletion, seizure disorder, GT dependence and recurrent aspiration pneumonias. He had a history of two to three admissions per year for respiratory infections. Because of the frequency of hospital admissions and frequent antibiotic courses, providers were concerned for posterior drooling and a salivagram was obtained. This showed aspiration of tracer into the trachea and bilateral bronchi. He had been maintained on glycopyrronium bromide (0.06mg/kg) TID without improvement in his symptoms. His TDS score was a 5 (constant drooling, always wet).

Otolaryngology was consulted to consider further interventions of botulinum toxin injections vs surgical interventions. The family was interested in the least invasive option and onabotulinumtoxinA injections were discussed. Given his young age of 5 years,

Otolaryngology agreed and was reluctant to start with surgical treatment. The decision was made to pursue parotid and submandibular gland onabotulinumtoxinA injections using ultrasound guidance with 20 units per submandibular gland and 25 units per parotid gland.

At 6-week follow-up Nathan was doing well with resolution of anterior drooling and no need for suctioning. His TDS score was 1. The family was concerned for slightly thicker secretions and glycopyrronium bromide was weaned. He continued to have improvement through 16 weeks when he was re-evaluated after a re-admission for aspiration pneumonia and the family had noted increased coughing and choking on secretions.

Treatment options included repeat onabotulinumtoxinA injections vs a surgical procedure. Given that he had responded so well the family preferred repeat onabotulinumtoxinA injections. These were performed 7 months following the initial injection at the same dose. Following repeat injections his TDS score has remained a 1 and his secretions have been minimal through 8-month follow-up. Complication after the second injections included xerostomia managed with mouth swabs.

Take-home points:

1. *Botulinum toxin injections are an effective management option for patients with anterior and/or posterior drooling.*

2. *The response can be variable, as exhibited by Nathan who had a favourable response on both occasions, but a more robust response following the second injection with continued improvement 8 months postoperatively.*

REFERENCES

Addy V, McElnay JC, Eyre DG et al. (1983) Risk factors in phenytoin-induced gingival hyperplasia. *J Periodontol* 54(6): 373–377.

Arvedson J, Clark H, Lazarus C, Schooling T, Frymark T (2010) The effects of oral-motor exercises on swallowing in children: an evidence-based systematic review. *Dev Med Child Neurol* 52(11): 1000–1013.

Bothwell JE, Clarke K, Dooley JM et al. (2002) Botulinum toxin A as a treatment for excessive drooling in children. *Pediatr Neurol* 27(1): 18–22.

Botti Rodrigues dos Santos MT, Masiero D, Ferreira Novo N, Lorenzetti Simionato MR (2003) Oral conditions in children with cerebral palsy. *J Dent Child* 70: 40–46.

Botti Rodrigues dos Santos MT, Souza CB (2009) Traumatic dental injuries in individuals with cerebral palsy. *Dent Traumatol* 25(3): 290–294.

Botti Rodrigues dos Santos MT, de Carvalho Batista R, Oliveira Guare R et al. (2011) Salivary osmolality and hydration status in children with cerebral palsy. *J Oral Pathol Med* 40: 582–586.

Camp-Bruno JA, Winsberg BG, Green-Parsons AR, Abrams JP (1989) Efficacy of benztropine therapy for drooling. *Dev Med Child Neurol* 31: 309–319.

Chauncey HH, Muench ME, Karpu KK, Wayler AH (1984) The effect of the loss of teeth on diet and nutrition. *Int Dent J* 34(2): 98–104.

Corrêa-Faria P, Martins CC, Bonecker M et al. (2016) Clinical factors and socio-demographic characteristics associated with dental trauma in children: a systematic review and meta-analysis. *Dent Traumatol* 32(5): 367–378.

Dias BL, Fernandes AR, Maia Filho HS (2016) Sialorrhea in children with cerebral palsy. *J Pediatr (Rio J)* 92(6) Nov–Dec: 549–558. PMID: 27281791.

Dias BLS, Fernandes AR, Maia Filho HS (2017) Treatment of drooling with sublingual atropine sulfate in children and adolescents with cerebral palsy. *Arquivos de Neuro-Psiquiatria* 75(5): 282–287. doi: 10.1590/0004-282x20170033.

Diéguez-Pérez M, de Nova-Garcia MJ, Mourelle-Martínez R, Bartolomé-Villar B (2016) Oral health in children with physical (cerebral palsy) and intellectual (Down syndrome) disabilities: Systemic review I. *J Clin Exp Dent* 8(3): e337–343.

Franklin DL, Luther F, Curzon MEJ (1996) The prevalence of malocclusion in children with cerebral palsy. *Eu J Orth* 18: 637–643.

Hegde AM, Shetty YR, Chandra Pani S (2008) Drooling of saliva and its effect on the oral health Status of children with cerebral palsy. *J Clin Ped Dent* 32(3): 235–238.

Jawadi AH, Casamassimo PS, Griffen A, Enrile B, Marcone M (2004) Comparison of oral findings in special needs children with and without gastrostomy. *Pediatr Dent* 26(3): 283–288.

Jongerius PH, van den Hoogen FJ, van Limbeek J, Gabreels FJ, van Hulst K, Rotteveel JJ (2004) Effect of botulinum toxin in the treatment of drooling: a controlled clinical trial. *Pediatrics* 114(3): 620–627. doi: 10.154/peds.2003-1104-L.

Khan WU, Campisi P, Nadarajah S et al. (2011) Botulinum toxin A for treatment of sialorrhea in children: an effective, minimally invasive approach. *Archives of Otolaryngol Head Neck Surg* 137(4): 339–344.

Lungren MP, Halula S, Coyne S, Sidell D, Racadio JM, Patel MN (2016) Ultrasound-guided botulinum toxin type A salivary gland injection in children for refractory sialorrhea: 10-year experience at a large tertiary children's hospital. *Pediatr Neurol* 54: 70–75.

Macedo CR, Silva AB, Machado MA et al. (2007) Occlusal splints for treating sleep bruxism (tooth grinding). *Cochrane Database Syst Rev* Oct 17 (4): CD005514.

Macedo C, Macedo E, Torloni MR et al. (2014) Pharmacotherapy for sleep bruxism. *Cochrane Database Syst Rev* Oct 23 (10): CD005578.

Manzano FS, Granero LM, Masiero D, dos Maria TB (2004) Treatment of muscle spasticity in patients with cerebral palsy using BTX-A: a pilot study. *Spec Care Dentist* 24(4): 235–239.

Martin TJ, Conley SF (2007) Long-term efficacy of intra-oral surgery for sialorrhea. *Otolaryngol Head Neck Surg* 137: 54–58.

Martinez-Mihi V, Silvestra FJ, Orellana LM, Silvestre-Rangil J (2014) Resting position of the head and malocclusion in a group of patients with cerebral palsy. *J Clin Exp Dent* 6(1): e1–6.

Miamoto CB, Ramos-Jorge ML, Pereira LJ, Paiva SM, Pordeus I, Marques LS (2010) Severity of malocclusion in patients with cerebral palsy: determinant factors. *Am J Orth Dentofac Orthoped* 138 (4) 394.e1–394.e5.

Mier RJ, Bachrach SJ, Lakin RC, Barker T, Childs J, Moran M (2000) Treatment of sialorrhea with glycopyrrolate: a double blind, dose-ranging study. *Arch Pediatr Adolesc Med* 154: 1214–1218.

Norderyd J, Graf J, Marcusson A et al. (2017) Sublingual administration of atropine eyedrops in children with excessive drooling – a pilot study. *Int J Paediatr Dent* 27: 22–29. doi: 10.1111/ipd.12219.

Norwood KW Jr, Slayton RL, Council on Children with Disabilities, Section on Oral Health (2013) Oral health care for children with developmental disabilities. *Pediatrics* 131(3) March: 614–619.

Ortega AO, Dos Santos MT, Mendes FM, Ciamponi AL (2014) Association between anticonvulsant drugs and teeth-grinding in children and adolescents with cerebral palsy. *J Oral Rehab* 41(9): 653–658.

Parr JR, Weldon E, Pennington L et al. (2014) The drooling reduction intervention trial (DRI): a single blind trial comparing the efficacy of glycopyrronium and hyoscine on drooling in children with neutralizability. *Trials* 15(1): 60. doi: 10.1186/1745-6215-15-60.

Parr JR, Todhunter E, Pennington L et al. (2018) Drooling Reduction Intervention randomised trial (DRI): comparing the efficacy and acceptability of hyoscine patches and glycopyrronium liquid on drooling in children with neurodisability. *Arch Dis Child* 103: 371–376.

Ranjitkar S, Kaidonis JA, Smales RJ (2012) Gastroesophageal reflux disease and tooth erosion. *Int J Dent* 479850. doi: 10.1155/2012/479850.

Reed J, Mans CK, Brietzke SE (2009) Surgical management of drooling: a meta-analysis. *Otolaryngol Head Neck Surg* 135(9): 924–931.

Reid SM, Johnstone BR, Westbury C, Rawicki B, Reddihough DS (2008) Randomized trial of botulinum toxin injections into the salivary glands to reduce drooling in children with neurological disorders. *Dev Med Child Neurol* 50(2): 123–128.

Scheffer AR, Erasmus C, van Hulst K, van Limbeek J, Jongerius PH, van den Hoogen FJ (2010) Efficacy and duration of botulinum toxin treatment for drooling in 131 children. *Otalaryngol Head Neck Surg* 136(9): 873–877.

Sjogreen L, Gonzalez Lindh M, Brodén M et al. (2018) Oral sensory-motor intervention for children and adolescents (3–18 years) with dysphagia or impaired saliva control secondary to congenital or early-acquired disabilities: a review of the literature, 2000 to 2016. *Ann Ot Rhin Laryn* 127(12): 978–985.

Souki BQ, Pimenta GB, Souki MQ, Franco LP, Becker HMG, Pinto JA (2009)) First permanent molar: first indicator of dental caries activity in initial mixed dentition. *Int J Pediatr Otorhinolaryngol* 73: 767–773.

Stamataki S, Behar P, Brodsky L (2008) Surgical management of drooling: clinical and caregiver satisfaction outcomes. *Int J Pediatr Otorhinolaryngol* 72: 1801–1805.

Van der Burg JJW, Didden R, Jongerius PH, Rotteveel JJ (2007) A descriptive analysis of studies on behavioural treatment of drooling (1970–2005). *Dev Med Child Neurol* 49: 390–394.

Wriedt S, Buhl V, Al-Nawas B, Wehrbein H (2009) Combined treatment of open bite – long term evaluation and relapse factors. *J Orofac Orthop* 70(4): 318–326.

Zeller RS, Lee HM, Cavanaugh PF, Davidson J (2012) Randomized Phase III evaluation of the efficacy and safety of novel glycopyrrolate oral solution for the management of chronic severe drooling in children with cerebral palsy or other neurologic conditions. *Ther Clin Risk Man* 8: 15–23.

CHAPTER 4

Gastrointestinal Problems in Children with Neurodisability: Causes, Symptoms and Management

Ilse Broekaert

INTRODUCTION

> **Case Study**
>
> *A 4-year-old girl with neurodegenerative disease is referred to our Paediatric Gastroenterology Clinic by her speech therapist because of feeding difficulties. Her parents suspect problems swallowing because of tonsillar hypertrophy and tonsillectomy is planned. She has always been small for her age, and for the last 6 months she is slowly falling off from her weight-for-age curve. She is already on lactulose because of constipation. Her neurologist started her on inhalational therapy consisting of salbutamol and fluticasone as well as on esomeprazole because of recurrent bronchitis. She is not vomiting. If she is not gaining weight after her tonsillectomy we will suggest hypercaloric feeds and after investigations possibly consider feeding via nasogastric tube or ultimately via percutaneous gastrostomy or even jejunal feeding if indicated.*

Gastrointestinal problems are encountered in more than 90% of children with neurological impairment (Del Giudice et al. 1999). Neurological impairment is a heterogeneous group of neurological disorders, which primarily relate to the central nervous system affecting speech, vision, motor skills, memory and learning disabilities. Diffuse brain lesions may disrupt neural modulation of gastrointestinal motility altering the flow of information from the cortex to the enteric nervous system leading to significant dysfunction in the gastrointestinal tract (Del Giudice et al. 1999; Quitadamo et al. 2016). The degree of gastrointestinal dysmotility correlates with the degree of damage to the developing central nervous system (Del Giudice et al. 1999). These underlying problems may be further complicated by other interacting factors (Fig. 4.1).

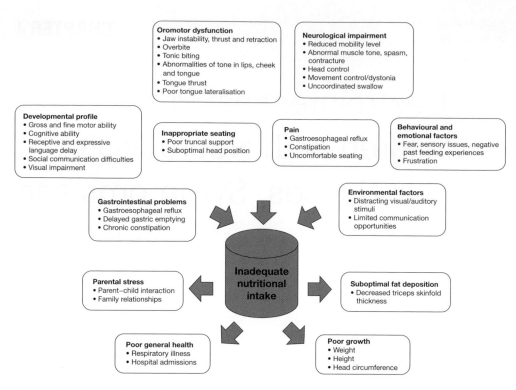

Oromotor dysfunction
- Jaw instability, thrust and retraction
- Overbite
- Tonic biting
- Abnormalities of tone in lips, cheek and tongue
- Tongue thrust
- Poor tongue lateralisation

Neurological impairment
- Reduced mobility level
- Abnormal muscle tone, spasm, contracture
- Head control
- Movement control/dystonia
- Uncoordinated swallow

Developmental profile
- Gross and fine motor ability
- Cognitive ability
- Receptive and expressive language delay
- Social communication difficulties
- Visual impairment

Inappropriate seating
- Poor truncal support
- Suboptimal head position

Pain
- Gastroesophageal reflux
- Constipation
- Uncomfortable seating

Behavioural and emotional factors
- Fear, sensory issues, negative past feeding experiences
- Frustration

Gastrointestinal problems
- Gastroesophageal reflux
- Delayed gastric emptying
- Chronic constipation

Environmental factors
- Distracting visual/auditory stimuli
- Limited communication opportunities

Parental stress
- Parent–child interaction
- Family relationships

Inadequate nutritional intake

Suboptimal fat deposition
- Decreased triceps skinfold thickness

Poor general health
- Respiratory illness
- Hospital admissions

Poor growth
- Weight
- Height
- Head circumference

Figure 4.1 Causal relationships between factors contributing to feeding difficulties and growth and general health in children with neurological impairment. (Reproduced from Andrew et al. 2012 with permission from BMJ Publishing Group Ltd.)

Gastrointestinal problems include oropharyngeal dysfunction, gastroesophageal reflux, delayed gastric emptying and constipation, and affect quality of life and nutritional status. Oropharyngeal dysfunction and gastroesophageal reflux disease predispose to pulmonary aspiration leading to recurrent respiratory infections, which is the most common cause of death in this population (Capriati et al. 2015).

Epilepsy occurs in more than 40% of children with neurological impairment and is associated with a disadvantageous prognosis as it can impede psychomotor development resulting in secondary changes to the central nervous system (Otapowicz et al. 2010). Symptoms such as drooling and gastroesophageal reflux may be aggravated by epilepsy, especially by frequent seizures and long-term pharmacotherapy (Otapowicz et al. 2010).

There is a strong association between the presence of oropharyngeal dysfunction and malnutrition (Campanozzi et al. 2007). Regular nutritional assessment will aid in identifying gastrointestinal problems, which are aggravated by neurological impairment such as cognitive disability, poor head control and truncal support, abnormal muscle tone and reduced mobility in these children (Fig. 4.1).

DYSPHAGIA/OROPHARYNGEAL DYSFUNCTION

Introduction and Definition

Oropharyngeal dysfunction (OPD) is present in 90% of children with neurological impairment and is a major risk factor for morbidity and mortality in this population (Reilly et al. 1996; Benfer et al. 2012). In The International Classification of Functioning, Disability and Health OPD is defined as impairment to the ingestion functions related to taking in and manipulating solids or liquids through the mouth into the body (Benfer et al. 2012). OPD encompasses impairment to any component of the oral-preparatory (sucking, munching, chewing and bolus formation), the oral (propulsive) (moving the food or fluid posteriorly through the oral cavity with the tongue into the back of the throat) and/or the pharyngeal phase of swallowing (swallowing the food or fluid and moving it through the pharynx to the oesophagus) that are associated with eating, drinking or controlling saliva (Morgan et al. 2012; van den Engel-Hoek et al. 2014). In neurologically impaired children solid boluses are managed more easily than liquid boluses and small liquid boluses more easily than large liquid boluses (Casas et al. 1994).

As 50% of OPD in children between 18–24 months of age resolves by 60 months, with improvement most common in children with Gross Motor Function Classification System (GMFCS) I–II, it is better to speak of delayed than disordered feeding abilities in a subgroup of these children (Benfer et al. 2017). Even orally fed children can have severe swallowing deficits (Bader & Niemann 2010) and those assessed to have normal oromotor skills may continue to demonstrate coughing during mealtimes until 6 years of age, suggesting a later maturation of the swallowing process (Benfer et al. 2015a).

Causes

The underlying swallowing problem in cerebral palsy is complex and is associated with abnormal control of swallowing, whereas in neuromuscular disorders it is mainly due to muscle weakness (van den Engel-Hoek et al. 2014). Deficits in the different levels of central and peripheral nervous system necessary for initiating, coordinating and modulating the swallowing process can result in dysphagia in one or all phases of swallowing (Engel et al. 1999).

The origin of OPD in cerebral palsy lies in the persistence of primitive reflexes, which hamper the development of physiological swallowing leading to absent or inefficient swallowing with a reduced mobility of the pharynx (Bader & Niemann 2010). This in turn leads to inadequate triggering of the swallowing reflex and a high risk for aspiration (Bader & Niemann 2010). OPD can also induce significant bonding problems between mother and child (Bader & Niemann 2010).

In addition to nervous system dysfunction, an unstable pelvis and trunk leading to poor head and neck positioning can reduce the ability for controlled oropharyngeal movements (Benfer et al. 2015a). Poor head position has also been related to a compromised airway protection by opening the airway, and the influence of gravity on flow rate of foods or fluids swallowed (Benfer et al. 2015a).

Symptoms

OPD should be considered in all neurologically impaired children even in the absence of obvious clinical signs and symptoms (Romano et al. 2017). OPD leads to the inability to consume sufficient food and fluids safely and is associated with prolonged mealtimes, poor growth and nutrition, and respiratory consequences from oropharyngeal aspiration. The most common signs on direct assessment are coughing (45%), multiple swallows (25%), a gurgly voice (23%), wet breathing (19%) and gagging (11%) (Benfer et al. 2015a).

The manifestation of malocclusion in this population has been attributed to the low tonicity of facial muscles and the uncoordinated movements of the lips and tongue (Miamoto et al. 2010). Overjet and an anterior open bite were significantly more prevalent in children with cerebral palsy (Miamoto et al. 2010). There is also a greater incidence of gingival problems, tooth caries, especially in the deciduous dentition, and tooth loss among children with cerebral palsy (Miamoto et al. 2010). These dental problems are described in greater detail in Chapter 3.

Additional feeding problems include a delayed or absent tongue lateralisation, persistent tongue thrust, and trunk instability resulting in problems with positioning for feeding (Chigira et al. 1994; Clancy & Hustad 2011).

Gross motor function is the best predictor of OPD (Benfer et al. 2016). Thus, 99% of children with GMFCS IV–V have dysphagia, and this is underestimated by parents (Calis et al. 2008). However, children with GMFCS I should also be monitored closely and, if indicated, have access to oral sensorimotor treatments (Benfer et al. 2017). There was a substantial discrepancy between the prolonged mealtimes reported by mothers and those actually observed at home (Reilly et al. 1996). Swallowing problems are frequently accompanied by dysarthria symptoms, which are especially severe when dysphagia involves the oral and pharyngeal phases (Otapowicz et al. 2010). Improvement of swallowing dysfunction has been mainly observed when only the oral phase of swallowing is affected (Otapowicz et al. 2010).

Oropharyngeal **aspiration** is defined as food or fluid entering the trachea and is present in up to 68% of severely neurologically impaired children (Mirrett et al. 1994). When problems in the pharyngeal or oesophageal phases of swallowing are suspected, imaging diagnostic techniques should be used to assess the risk of aspiration (Calis et al. 2008). If there are more significant neurological lesions there is a higher rate of silent aspirations. The presence of drooling is a warning sign for aspiration of saliva and food (Bader & Niemann 2010). However, clinical signs such as wet voice, wet breathing and cough have only a 33–67% sensitivity to predict aspiration of liquids on videofluoroscopy (Noll et al. 2011).

Investigations

Thorough evaluation and intensive management of feeding difficulties are often deferred until neurologically impaired children are medically or nutritionally compromised (Mirrett et al. 1994). However, early screening and diagnostic work-up may improve growth and nutritional outcomes and prevent malnutrition and chronic aspiration.

The mainstay of evaluating OPD is the direct **observation** of mealtimes with the optional use of standardised and validated scoring systems (Romano et al. 2017). Scores obtained by tests such as the Oral Motor Assessment Scale, the Schedule for Oral Motor Assessment, the Eating and Drinking Ability Classification System and the Exeter Dysphagia Assessment Technique provide valid and reliable systems for classifying eating and drinking performance and help to identify areas of dysfunction contributing to feeding difficulties (Reilly et al. 1995; Selley et al. 2000; Ortega Ade et al. 2009; Sellers et al. 2014).

Videofluoroscopy remains one of the key investigations and is the criterion standard for penetration or aspiration of food, especially if fibreoptic endoscopy (see below) remains inconclusive (Buckler 2016; Romano et al. 2017). Based on videofluoroscopic findings recommendations such as changes in body and head position and consistency of food and of feeding techniques can be made leading to improvements in mealtime behaviour with reduced coughing and choking (Griggs et al. 1989). Thus, in the reclined position with the neck flexed, there is a reduction in aspiration and possibly in oral leakage as well as a possible improvement in retention (Larnert & Ekberg 1995). However, in children with difficulties in the pharyngeal phase (e.g. upper oesophageal sphincter spasm) feeding is best in the erect position (Morton et al. 1993).

Fibreoptic endoscopic evaluation of swallowing (FEES) is a low-cost, rather well-tolerated and repeatable investigation that can be performed in neurologically impaired children as young as a few days old. It detects potentially dangerous penetration or aspiration of saliva, fluid or food (Beer et al. 2014). FEES enables the physician to change airway and feeding management especially in children who formerly have been fed orally without suspicion of (severe) swallowing deficits (Bader & Niemann 2010). It does not directly prove food aspiration (Bockler 2016). It detects more aspiration than clinical assessment, but it is an artificial situation necessitating competency and training by a multidisciplinary team (Beer et al. 2014; Reynolds et al. 2016). The advantages of fibreoptic endoscopy are the lack of radiation exposure and administration of barium, the possibilities to position the child and its high safety and reliability (Bader & Niemann 2010; Beer et al. 2014).

Impedance measurements study the movement of liquids and air in the oesophagus and can detect acid and non-acid reflux. In neurologically impaired children impedance studies evaluate the pharyngeal swallow and can predict deglutitive aspiration risks (Noll et al. 2011).

During **high-resolution manometry**, the pharyngeal contractility, the upper oesophageal sphincter tone and relaxation during swallowing is measured. It can be performed in conjunction with fluoroscopy, but reference values from typically developing infants and children are needed for interpretation (Rommel et al. 2006).

Electromyography of the pharyngeal muscles is a non-invasive diagnostic method that evaluates the pharyngeal phase of swallowing and that is applicable to children above 5 years (Ozdemirkiran et al. 2007). Through electromyography the maximal volume of a single swallow by progressively increasing water volumes can be measured. It may be used as a screening test before invasive tests such as videofluoroscopy and/or fibreoptic endoscopy are applied (Ozdemirkiran et al. 2007).

Ultrasound imaging can provide useful information with regard to the oral cavity and the soft tissue structures by capturing the salient features of tongue/hyoid/palate activity and bolus transport across the tongue and through the hypopharyngeal area (Yang et al. 1997). Kenny et al. were able to demonstrate a lack of control of the posterior part of the tongue in many neurologically impaired children (Kenny et al. 1989).

Upper gastrointestinal endoscopy is not routinely used in neurologically impaired children to assess for OPD.

Management

Treatment of OPD ideally involves an appropriately skilled multidisciplinary team (speech and language therapy, psychology, orthopaedics, orthodontics, paediatrics, neurology, nutrition) beginning at an early age (Miamoto et al. 2010; Romano et al. 2017).

Speech and language therapy often forms the mainstay of treatment of OPD in neurologically impaired children (Romano et al. 2017). If possible and safe enough the aim should be to optimise oral feeding. In a significant proportion of neurologically impaired children, management will aim to modify time allocated to feeding, improve posture and adapt feed consistency to limit complications such as aspiration (Romano et al. 2017). Pureed foods and fluids are likely to be more efficiently eaten by children with lower gross motor function (Benfer et al. 2015b). However, fluids are most associated with OPD thus increasing the risk of aspiration (Benfer et al. 2015b). Oral sensorimotor therapy aims at improving the individual and combined functioning of lips, cheeks, tongue and pharyngeal structures. In a systematic review of speech therapy techniques in rehabilitation, 64% use oral sensorimotor therapy as a therapeutic method, 36% report continuing education as a therapeutic approach and only 18% and 9% use the Bobath and the Castillo Morales concepts, respectively (Hirata & Santos 2012).

Oral sensorimotor therapy leads to significant improvement in spoon feeding, chewing and swallowing, but not in drinking skills. Despite these improvements, however, there is no evidence that such oral sensorimotor treatment is effective in the restoration of a normal nutritional state (Gisel 1996). The children's growth must be monitored carefully and early (oral) caloric supplementation may provide necessary energy for growth (Gisel 1996; Romano et al. 2017). Tracheoesophageal diversion and laryngotracheal separation can prevent aspiration pneumonia, decrease morbidity of children with severe neurological impairment and improve the quality of life of parents and family (Takano et al. 2015).

GASTROESOPHAGEAL REFLUX

Introduction and Definition

Neurologically impaired children are at a particularly high risk for gastroesophageal reflux disease (GORD) with a reported incidence as high as 70% (Reyes et al. 1993; Bohmer et al. 1997; Del Giudice et al. 1999; Vandenplas et al. 2009; Bayram et al. 2016). GORD is attributed to a motility disturbance affecting the oesophagus and the lower oesophageal sphincter mechanism, and leads to retrograde, involuntary, effortless regurgitation of gastric contents into the oesophagus (Vernon-Roberts & Sullivan 2013).

Causes

The pathophysiological mechanisms of GORD are multifactorial (Vernon-Roberts & Sullivan 2013). Motor pattern generators localised in the central nervous system play a key role in controlling oesophageal peristalsis and lower oesophageal sphincter activity (Tambucci et al. 2015). The presence of low impedance values in the oesophagus reflects oesophageal motor abnormalities (Tambucci et al. 2015). Children with cerebral palsy are likely to have a low resting tone of the lower oesophageal sphincter (Turk et al. 2013). The neurological damage may cause poor self-protective mechanisms and oesophageal dysmotility with decreased appetite, abnormal swallowing and an increased gag reflex. In addition, delayed gastric emptying with delayed oesophageal clearance, skeletal abnormalities such as scoliosis, abnormal sensory integration, abnormal tone of the abdominal musculature, constipation, obesity and seizures can all cause increased abdominal pressure increasing reflux frequency (Reyes et al. 1993; Bohmer et al. 1997; Vandenplas et al. 2009; Vernon-Roberts & Sullivan 2013; Tambucci et al. 2015).

Retching is the laboured rhythmic activity of the diaphragm and the anterior abdominal wall musculature and is the first part of the emetic reflex. It needs to be differentiated from gastroesophageal reflux (Sullivan 2008). In children with neurological impairment the emetic reflex may be hypersensitive or there may be loss of its physiological inhibition (Sullivan 2008).

Medication such as anticholinergics and sedatives, which are frequently prescribed for neurologically impaired children, decrease the lower oesophageal sphincter tone favouring GORD (Bohmer et al. 1997).

Because of their often profound physical disabilities, many children spend long periods in the supine position, thus minimising the effect of gravity to aid oesophageal clearance (Vernon-Roberts & Sullivan 2013).

There is a significant, unexplained association with the male sex, but poor nutritional status alone seems not be associated with GORD (Reyes et al. 1993). Hiatal hernia is not necessary for the development of GORD or oesophagitis, but is found to be a major risk factor (Bohmer et al. 1997).

Early onset neurological impairment implicating more severe neurological sequelae, abnormal EEG results, and mitochondrial disease are risk factors for severe GORD (Kim et al. 2017). An abnormal EEG can be considered a risk factor for GORD, but seizure activity does not aggravate GORD directly (Kim et al. 2017). Rather, abnormal brain function itself most likely affects reflux activity (Kim et al. 2017).

Symptoms

Symptoms such as vomiting, haematemesis, rumination and regurgitation are indicative for GORD (Bohmer et al. 1997). Despite its high incidence, GORD in neurologically impaired children is difficult to recognise as the symptoms are non-specific and many children cannot precisely express their symptoms (Kim et al. 2017). Atypical presentations with anxiety, depressive symptoms, automutilation, food refusal, restlessness, apparent seizures and dystonia are frequent (Bohmer et al. 1997; Vandenplas et al. 2009). Chronic obstructive pulmonary disease or other respiratory complications, failure to thrive and a poor growth and nutritional state, iron deficiency and anaemia may also be related to GORD (Gustafsson & Tibbling 1994; Bohmer et al. 1997). Severe grades of GORD with Barrett's oesophagus, peptic strictures and upper gastrointestinal haemorrhage can be seen in this young patient population (Bohmer et al. 1997). Unfortunately, diagnosis of GORD is often delayed until significant oesophagitis or potentially fatal aspiration pneumonia occurs (Kim et al. 2017). In neurologically impaired children there is a relatively high prevalence of *Helicobacter pylori* infection which may cause loss of appetite, abdominal discomfort, reflux symptoms and weight loss, and so forth; however, only rarely have duodenal ulcers been found (Bohmer et al. 1997).

Retching must be distinguished from the relatively effortless gastroesophageal reflux as it is characterised by forceful vomiting. Episodes of retching are characterised by a prodrome of salivation, tachycardia, peripheral vasoconstriction and nausea possibly leading to emesis (Sullivan 2008). Retching also persists after fundoplication and may even drive the wrap at the gastroesophageal junction through the diaphragm leading to failure of fundoplication (Richards et al. 2001).

Sandifer syndrome (spasmodic torsional dystonia with arching of the back and opisthotonic posturing, mainly involving the neck and back) is an uncommon but specific manifestation of GORD, which can mimic epileptic seizures without concomitant ictal EEG changes (Vandenplas et al. 2009; Bayram et al. 2016). The mechanisms of these involuntary reflex movements in Sandifer syndrome are unclear, although it is considered that the abnormal movements during reflux protect the airways from reflux material (Bayram et al. 2016). The dystonic movements may also be triggered by the abdominal discomfort caused by gastroesophageal reflux and oesophagitis (Bayram et al. 2016). It may not always resolve with antireflux treatment (Vandenplas et al. 2009; Bayram et al. 2016). GORD can also cause laryngospasm, bradycardia and apnoeic episodes in infants, which might be mistaken for epileptic seizures (Bayram et al. 2016).

Rumination is the deliberate regurgitation of food into the mouth followed in part by emesis, rechewing and repeated swallowing. It is most often found in neurologically impaired children. The cause of rumination can be over- and understimulation from parents and caregivers, seeking self-gratification and seeking self-stimulus due to the lack or abundance of external stimuli. It differs from rumination in normally developed children as it is present both day and night and not only after a meal (Bohmer et al. 1997). Therefore, in neurologically impaired children, rumination causes much more damage because these children not only ruminate food (with a normal pH), but most of the time gastric fluid with a very low pH with the potential to induce oesophageal damage (Bohmer et al. 1997).

Superior mesenteric artery syndrome is a rare cause of proximal intestinal obstruction occurring due to compression of the duodenum between the aorta and the superior mesenteric artery (Neuman et al. 2014). It is typically due to loss of the mesenteric fat pad surrounding the superior mesenteric artery as a result of malnutrition. Duodenal obstruction is dependent on the child's position and may be partially relieved with insufflation during oesophagogastroduodenoscopy (Neuman et al. 2014). Symptoms include abdominal pain, nausea, early satiety, vomiting and further weight loss (Neuman et al. 2014). Conservative measures including nasogastric tube decompression, correction of underlying electrolyte abnormalities and increased nutritional support are necessary to alleviate the symptoms (Neuman et al. 2014). In order to reverse malnutrition temporary jejunal tube feeding which bypasses the duodenal obstruction may be performed. However, when conservative methods fail surgical options may be necessary (Neuman et al. 2014).

Dumping syndrome is caused by a too rapid passage of often undigested food and liquid into the duodenum (Sullivan 2008). It is a common complication after fundoplication because of elevated gastric pressure causing increased gastric emptying, especially when a pyloroplasty has been performed (Bufler et al. 2001). Common symptoms are decreased appetite, postprandial nausea, retching, tachycardia, pallor, lethargy and watery diarrhoea (Ukleja 2005). Treatment consists of feeding complex carbohydrates to inhibit gastric emptying and decrease reactive hypoglycaemia and, if that fails, continuous intragastric feeding (Sullivan 2008).

Investigations

Given the high prevalence of GORD, a therapeutic trial of proton pump inhibitors with careful clinical follow-up is an acceptable management if the provisional diagnosis of GORD is reached by clinical history in this clinically fragile group of children (Romano et al. 2017).

Upper gastrointestinal endoscopy is the method of choice to evaluate for oesophageal damage and biopsies are necessary to identify other causes of oesophagitis and to diagnose and monitor Barrett's oesophagus (Vandenplas et al. 2009; Romano et al. 2017). Lower oesophageal pH studies can quantify oesophageal acidic exposure and in combination with multichannel intraluminal impedance can also detect weakly acidic and non-acidic reflux episodes (Vandenplas et al. 2009; Romano et al. 2017). In patients with suspicion of gastroparesis or gastric outlet obstruction barium contrast studies should be performed (Vandenplas et al. 2009; Romano et al. 2017).

Management

Treatment of GORD in children consists of lifestyle changes, pharmacological therapies and surgical treatment.

LIFESTYLE CHANGES

Changes in feeding volume, consistency and frequency may be helpful, as may positional changes and control of muscular spasticity.

Thickening of formula by pectin partially decreased gastroesophageal reflux as measured by oesophageal pH monitoring, and can improve vomiting and respiratory symptoms in children with neurological impairment (Miyazawa et al. 2008). The viscosity of formula increases approximately 70-fold by the low-pectin and 180-fold by the high-pectin diet changing the liquid into a semi-solid meal (Miyazawa et al. 2008). Pectin also decreased the number of infant regurgitation episodes and improved bowel movements; it tended to decrease respiratory symptoms such as cough or wheeze, and the frequency of oxygen use for dyspnoea (Miyazawa et al. 2008). Furthermore, pectin delayed gastric emptying and increased satiety in obese individuals; however, low concentrations of pectin liquid did not cause delayed gastric emptying, and even decreased gastric residue, which might have been because pectin improved bowel motility (Miyazawa et al. 2008). A high-pectin diet decreased the number of episodes of vomiting (Miyazawa et al. 2008). The adverse effects of pectin are on fat absorption and intestinal solubility or absorption of ferrous iron (Miyazawa et al. 2008).

In a group of exclusively gastrostomy-fed neurologically impaired children there was a significant reduction in episodes and duration of gastroesophageal reflux when consuming whey-based formula (Khoshoo et al. 1996). A 50% whey formula significantly reduced gagging and retching in children with severe neurological impairment (Fried et al. 1992).

Furthermore, malnutrition can be regarded as a risk factor for GORD and, therefore, intensification of feeding with a hypercaloric diet leads to a marked improvement of GORD (Campanozzi et al. 2007).

PHARMACOLOGICAL THERAPIES

Acid suppression drugs are the mainstay of treatment of GORD in neurologically impaired children (Vandenplas et al. 2009; Romano et al. 2017). Proton pump inhibitors are regarded as first-line treatment as they are superior to histamine-2 receptor antagonists (Vandenplas et al. 2009). Because of the considerable risk of complications with antireflux surgery, the use of proton pump inhibitor treatment is an appropriate and cost-effective means of managing long-term GORD in neurologically impaired children (Cheung et al. 2001; Vandenplas et al. 2009). When prolonged treatment is necessary, special attention should be given to side effects such as pulmonary and gastrointestinal infections and malabsorption of micronutrients. As objective diagnostic tests are the only reliable method to monitor for controlled GORD, periodical evaluation of long-term GORD therapy such as via pH impedance studies, oesophagogastroduodenoscopy or barium swallow studies under or after holding reflux treatment in children with neurological impairment is necessary (Romano et al. 2017).

Proton pump inhibitors do not affect the total number of reflux episodes; they only decrease the acidity of refluxate with a compensatory increase of the number of weakly acidic episodes (Turk et al. 2013). Nevertheless, the majority of children with typical reflux symptoms may report symptom improvement (Turk et al. 2013). The treatment of weakly acid and weakly alkaline reflux, however, remains a challenge (Turk et al. 2013). The suggested dosage of omeprazole is 1.0–2.3mg/kg/day (Cheung et al. 2001). Treatment duration of 3–6 months can lead to resolution of reflux oesophagitis and other reflux symptoms including vomiting, gastrointestinal bleeding and aspiration pneumonia (Cheung et al. 2001; Turk et al. 2013).

Proton pump inhibitors can also significantly reduce bile reflux into the oesophagus, and the proposed mechanism is a reduction of total reflux due to decreased gastric secretion and fluid content (Turk et al. 2013).

Baclofen at a dosage of 0.7mg/kg/day may be useful for reduction of vomiting, but care with regard to dosing and side effects is required (Kawai et al. 2004; Vandenplas et al. 2009). The efficacy and safety of other prokinetic drugs such as metoclopramide, domperidone, betanechol and erythromycin for GORD treatment in neurologically impaired children have not been studied, but their use may be considered in uncontrolled GORD (Romano et al. 2017).

SURGICAL TREATMENT

As for typically developed children, antireflux surgery may be of benefit in children with confirmed GORD who have failed optimal medical therapy, who are dependent on medical therapy over a long period of time, or who have significant complications of GORD (Romano et al. 2017). Children with respiratory complications may especially benefit from antireflux surgery. Fundoplication improves weight gain, chest infections, vomiting and feeding intolerance (O'Loughlin et al. 2013). However, neurologically impaired children have an increased risk for perioperative morbidity and mortality, postoperative failure and persistence/recurrence of GORD (Vernon-Roberts & Sullivan 2013). Fundoplication alters the gastroesophageal anatomy and function, and may lead to vagal nerve damage that sensitises the emetic reflex leading to gagging and retching (Vernon-Roberts & Sullivan 2013). Complications directly related to the surgery may include bloating, impaired gastric accommodation, gastric hypersensitivity, rapid gastric emptying or even dumping syndrome, gagging, retching or dysphagia (Vernon-Roberts & Sullivan 2013). Therefore, children whose symptoms are well controlled on medical therapy may not gain additional benefit from antireflux surgery. A common complication of gastrostomy placement is the worsening of gastroesophageal reflux (Vernon-Roberts & Sullivan 2013). This can also be caused by too aggressive intragastric feeding. However, a routine antireflux procedure should not be performed at the time of gastrostomy placement because of inherent increased morbidity (Romano et al. 2017).

Placement of a gastrojejunal tube is a reasonable alternative to fundoplication and gastrostomy for neurologically impaired children with GORD, refractory vomiting and retching (Wales et al. 2002). The majority can be inserted image-guided without general anaesthesia (Wales et al. 2002). This technique failed in only 8% of children, with the subsequent need for fundoplication (Wales et al. 2002). Of the children with gastrojejunostomy, 15% showed spontaneous improvement and had their jejunal feeding tube removed (Wales et al. 2002). In another study, there was a trend towards more major complications with fundoplication/gastrostomy (29%) compared to gastrojejunostomy (12%) (Livingston et al. 2015). Minor complications were more common with gastrojejunostomy (70%) than fundoplication/gastrostomy (45%), but this was also not statistically significant (Livingston et al. 2015). A major drawback of gastrojejunostomy is the requirement of a continuous feeding regimen (Livingston et al. 2015).

Total oesophagogastric disconnection and Roux-en-Y oesophagojejunostomy is an invasive but effective therapy for GORD in neurologically impaired children (Lansdale et al. 2015). This 'once-and-for-all' therapy should only be considered as definitive therapy in special and complex situations, for example children with severe neurological impairment necessitating repeated antireflux surgery or microgastria that cannot be treated with one of the gastric augmentation techniques (Kunisaki et al. 2011; Lansdale et al. 2015; Romano et al. 2017).

CHRONIC CONSTIPATION

Introduction and Definition

Constipation is a common problem, being present in 26–74% of neurologically impaired children, and 55% use laxatives (Del Giudice et al. 1999; Elawad & Sullivan 2001; Veugelers et al. 2010). All of the generally accepted definitions of functional constipation include elements that are not applicable to a neurologically impaired paediatric population (Veugelers et al. 2010). A suggested definition of constipation in children with neurological impairment is the presence of two or more of the following symptoms for at least 2 months: (1) two or fewer defecations per week, (2) painful or hard bowel movements, and (3) the presence of a large faecal mass in the abdomen (Veugelers et al. 2010).

Causes

Constipation is generally believed to be the result of both neurological and lifestyle factors (Veugelers et al. 2010). The enteric nervous system is modulated by a wide range of inputs from the central nervous system (Elawad & Sullivan 2001). Damage to the central nervous system is one of the most important risk factors for constipation, even when adjusted for potential confounding factors such as immobility or pain (Veugelers et al. 2010). Hypotonia, skeletal muscle incoordination, skeletal deformities and prolonged immobility exacerbate constipation and faecal incontinence. Constipation is significantly more common among children using medication known to slow intestinal motility and children with severe motor disabilities (GMFCS V) (Veugelers et al. 2010). Immobility with the inability to sit/squat on the toilet, and the lack of gravity, reduce the contribution from raised intra-abdominal pressure, and decrease the ability to stabilise the rectum (Elawad & Sullivan 2001).

In a study, dietary intakes of water and fibre were below the recommended amounts in 87% and 53% of children, respectively (Veugelers et al. 2010). The majority of enteral feeds are without fibre supplements. The relatively poor fluid intake is often due to fear about choking and aspiration (Elawad & Sullivan 2001). However, fluid and fibre intake did not correlate with defecation frequency or other symptoms of constipation (Veugelers et al. 2010).

A number of drugs such as anticholinergics and opiates have a negative effect on both small and large bowel intestinal transit time. Sodium valproate, phenothiazines, baclofen, glycopyrrolate and scopolamine are known to increase constipation (Elawad & Sullivan 2001). Aluminium-containing antacids, diuretics, antidepressants, antihistamines, antispasmodics, opioids and anticonvulsants were associated with a nearly two- to three-fold increased risk of constipation and, because they are in common use, can explain a relatively large number of cases (Talley et al. 2003).

Symptoms

A delayed passage of meconium (i.e. more than 24 hours after birth) indicating Hirschsprung disease should always be excluded.

A delay in diagnosing chronic constipation is a particular problem in children with neurological impairment either because it is accepted as an inevitable consequence of the neurological impairment or because a higher priority is given to other aspects of medical management such as treatment of seizures or postural deformity (Elawad & Sullivan 2001). Moreover, communication difficulties worsen delay and failure to recognise the problem as the neurologically impaired child is often unable to express the discomfort caused by constipation. The average duration of upper intestinal symptoms such as abdominal pain, GORD, nausea and vomiting secondary to chronic constipation is 16 months (Borowitz & Sutphen 2004). Furthermore, there is poor agreement between parents' recall of their child's bowel habits and stool frequency as assessed by prospective symptom diaries (Borowitz & Sutphen 2004).

The majority of children with idiopathic slow transit constipation have delayed gastric emptying and some of these children demonstrate retention of gastric solids and liquids up to 360 minutes after a meal that may prevent the change from the fed to fasted motility pattern in the stomach (Borowitz & Sutphen 2004). In a study, 26 of 34 had recurrent vomiting, six complained of chronic nausea, 17 had chronic symptoms of gastroesophageal reflux, and 20 complained of chronic or recurrent abdominal pain, most often in the epigastric region (Borowitz & Sutphen 2004). Smaller numbers experienced early satiety, choking, gagging, dysphagia or intermittent diarrhoea (Borowitz & Sutphen 2004). Chronic upper gastrointestinal symptoms rapidly and completely resolved when underlying constipation was treated (Borowitz & Sutphen 2004).

Because most children need to use diapers, faecal incontinence is difficult to discern from encopresis by obstipation and an enlarged rectum in children with neurological impairment (Elawad & Sullivan 2001; Veugelers et al. 2010). The aim of management in these children is to reduce the contribution of faecal incontinence by constipation.

Investigations

In children with neurological impairment, constipation may be diagnosed by a thorough history, an abdominal and perineal examination and if necessary a digital rectal examination and the appropriate diagnostic imaging (Romano et al. 2017).

Transabdominal ultrasound is a non-invasive and reliable method to assess the rectal filling state, and can replace digital rectal examination (Burgers et al. 2013). An excellent agreement was found between rectal diameter on ultrasound and rectal filling state as obtained by digital rectal examination, but there are no studies on neurologically impaired children (Burgers et al. 2013). In a study by Burgers et al. (2013), no linear correlation was found between age and rectal diameter on ultrasound. The rectal diameter is categorised as greater than 30mm (enlarged) and 30mm or less (normal); and the latter category is subcategorised as less than 25mm and 25–30mm (Burgers et al. 2013). An enlarged rectum can also be defined as having a rectopelvic ratio of more than 0.61 (Elawad & Sullivan 2001).

If the diagnosis is uncertain an abdominal radiograph may be helpful. The use of radio-opaque markers to assess colonic transit time is helpful to quantify constipation in those cases where management is difficult (Park et al. 2004; Veugelers et al. 2010). A transit time delay in the proximal colon was a dominant finding in constipated neurologically impaired children, suggesting that a disruption of the neural modulation of colon motility is responsible for constipation (Park et al. 2004). However, the prevalence of a transit time delay at the rectosigmoid colon implied that altered motor behaviour of the muscles of the recto-anal region might also contribute to the defecation problem (Park et al. 2004).

Management

In children with neurological impairment treatment of constipation should conform to the standard for typically developing children unless there is a risk of aspiration of polyethylene glycol (Romano et al. 2017).

If necessary, rectal disimpaction should be performed before starting maintenance therapy. This can be performed with rectal enemas (sodium citrate or sodium acid phosphate) or with a high dose of polyethylene glycol (1.5g/kg), as the application of enemas is often uncomfortable, for 3–6 consecutive days (Pashankar & Bishop 2001). Initial rectal disimpaction results in less faecal incontinence and prevents subsequent undertreatment (Burgers et al. 2013). If the child is distressed the enema can be administered under sedation (Elawad & Sullivan 2001). For a successful evacuation in a child with faecal loading beyond the rectum, however, rectal enema should be coupled with intestinal lavage with polyethylene glycol solution delivered via a nasogastric or a gastrostomy tube.

As a maintenance therapy, daily administration of polyethylene glycol at a mean dose of 0.8g/kg is effective and safe (Pashankar & Bishop 2001). Physicians tend to be prudent in prescribing laxatives in children with neurological impairment and the dosing is frequently inadequate (Veugelers et al. 2010). Polyethylene glycol acts as an osmotic agent, increasing faecal water content (Pashankar & Bishop 2001). The added electrolytes prevent faecal losses with large-volume lavage (Pashankar & Bishop 2001). However, electrolytes have an unpleasant salty taste, limiting compliance (Pashankar & Bishop 2001). Maintenance laxative therapy is often required for many months (Pashankar & Bishop 2001). The aim of the therapy is one to three soft–runny stools per day (Pashankar & Bishop 2001). Side effects of polyethylene glycol are transient dose-dependent diarrhoea and flatulence (Pashankar & Bishop 2001). Particular caution is advised in children with a high risk for aspiration (Veugelers et al. 2010) as aspiration of polyethylene glycol can be fatal. Unlike lactulose, polyethylene glycol is not fermentable by colonic bacterial flora and, therefore, does not cause gas production or acidic stools, avoiding abdominal discomfort and perianal irritation (Pashankar & Bishop 2001).

Magnesium hydroxide is a good long-term therapy, but compliance is often a problem because of its unpleasant taste (Pashankar & Bishop 2001). Mineral oil is a safe therapy except for the risk of aspiration in susceptible children and infants, and thus in those with an unsafe swallow its use is contraindicated (Pashankar & Bishop 2001). Stimulant laxatives such as senna, bisacodyl or sodium picosulphate are generally not recommended for long-term use in children as they may cause abdominal pain and melanosis coli due to anthraquinone in senna (Pashankar & Bishop 2001). In the case of anal fissures, improving perianal hygiene promotes healing and topical lignocaine lessens pain on defecation.

Increasing fluid and fibre intakes are additional strategies to treat constipation in neurologically impaired children (Romano et al. 2017). Fibre-containing formula increases stool size and improves stool consistency without increasing stool frequency (Fischer et al. 1985). Particular attention should be given to the child's fluid intake, especially when problems such as drooling and gastroesophageal reflux are present (Elawad & Sullivan 2001). Furthermore, abdominal massage of 20 minutes daily leads to an improved quality of life of neurologically impaired children with a relief in constipation symptoms in up to 88%, a reduction in laxative medication of 58%, an improved dietary intake of 41% and enhanced parent–child relationships (Bromley 2014).

In refractory cases, hydrocolonic enemas and antegrade continence enemas can successfully treat chronic constipation (Rodriguez et al. 2011). The antegrade continence enema (Malone procedure) is particularly successful in faecal incontinence, and has proved to be acceptable for both parents and children (Elawad & Sullivan 2001; King et al. 2005). The Chait button is well tolerated and safe and decreases the incidence of stomal stenosis, but is associated with increased granulation tissue (King et al. 2005). Perforation of the appendix is a serious complication (King et al. 2005). Laparoscopic-assisted percutaneous endoscopic caecostomy (LAPEC) is a safe, minimally invasive procedure for caecostomy placement in children with refractory constipation or faecal incontinence (Rodriguez et al. 2011). LAPEC provides both endoscopic and laparoscopic visualisation, thereby significantly decreasing the risk of pressure necrosis and skin breakdown from a button that is too tight or leakage from one that is too loose (Rodriguez et al. 2011).

Rarely, a defunctioning ileostomy or colostomy has to be placed for the management of extreme megacolon secondary to chronic constipation (Elawad & Sullivan 2001). The use of transcutaneous electrical stimulation using interferential current as a possible treatment requires further investigations (King et al. 2005).

SUMMARY

As portrayed above, gastrointestinal problems such as oropharyngeal dysfunction, gastroesophageal reflux and constipation are very frequent in neurologically impaired children. They not only affect quality of life, but also nutritional status and may predispose to recurrent respiratory infections. Gastrointestinal problems are under-recognised in neurologically impaired children, but a multidisciplinary approach involving paediatric neurology, paediatric gastroenterology, paediatric pulmonary, paediatric surgery, speech and language therapy, physiotherapy, psychology as well as a dietary team may lead to earlier diagnosis, more appropriate management and improved overall outcome.

REFERENCES

Andrew MJ, Parr JR, Sullivan PB (2012) Feeding difficulties in children with cerebral palsy. *Arch Dis Child-Ed Pract* 97: 222–229. doi: 10.1136/archdischild-2011-300914.

Bader CA, Niemann G (2010) Dysphagia in children with cerebral palsy – fiberoptic-endoscopic findings. *Laryngo Rhino Otologie* 89: 90–94. doi: 10.1055/s-0029-1237348.

Bayram AK, Canpolat M, Karacabey N et al. (2016) Misdiagnosis of gastroesophageal reflux disease as epileptic seizures in children. *Brain Dev* 38: 274–279. doi: 10.1016/j.braindev.2015.09.009.

Beer S, Hartlieb T, Muller A, Granel M, Staudt M (2014) Aspiration in children and adolescents with neurogenic dysphagia: comparison of clinical judgment and fiberoptic endoscopic evaluation of swallowing. *Neuropediatrics* 45: 402–405. doi: 10.1055/s-0034-1387814.

Benfer KA, Weir KA, Boyd RN (2012) Clinimetrics of measures of oropharyngeal dysphagia for preschool children with cerebral palsy and neurodevelopmental disabilities: a systematic review. *Dev Med Child Neurol* 54: 784–795. doi: 10.1111/j.1469-8749.2012.04302.x.

Benfer KA, Weir KA, Bell KL, Ware RS, Davies PS, Boyd RN (2015a) Clinical signs suggestive of pharyngeal dysphagia in preschool children with cerebral palsy. *Res Dev Dis* 38: 192–201. doi: 10.1016/j.ridd.2014.12.021.

Benfer KA, Weir KA, Bell KL, Ware RS, Davies PS, Boyd RN (2015b) Food and fluid texture consumption in a population-based cohort of preschool children with cerebral palsy: relationship to dietary intake. *Dev Med Child Neurol* 57: 1056–1063. doi: 10.1111/dmcn.12796.

Benfer KA, Weir KA, Bell KL, Ware RS, Davies PS, Boyd RN (2016) Longitudinal study of oropharyngeal dysphagia in preschool children with cerebral palsy. *Arch Phys Med Rehab* 97: 552–560.e9. doi: 10.1016/j.apmr.2015.11.016.

Benfer KA, Weir KA, Bell KL, Ware RS, Davies PSW, Boyd RN (2017) Oropharyngeal dysphagia and cerebral palsy. *Pediatrics* 140. doi: 10.1542/peds.2017-0731.

Bockler R (2016) FEES in infants with swallowing disorders – a feasible procedure? *Laryngo Rhino Otologie* 95: 192–196. doi: 10.1055/s-0035-1555886.

Bohmer CJ, Niezen de Boer MC, Klinkenberg-Knol EC et al. (1997) Gastroesophageal reflux disease in intellectually disabled individuals: leads for diagnosis and the effect of omeprazole therapy. *Am J Gastroenterol* 92: 1475–1479.

Borowitz SM, Sutphen JL (2004) Recurrent vomiting and persistent gastroesophageal reflux caused by unrecognized constipation. *Clin Pediatr (Phila)* 43: 461–466. doi: 10.1177/000992280404300507.

Bromley D (2014) Abdominal massage in the management of chronic constipation for children with disability. *Community Pract* 87: 25–29.

Bufler P, Ehringhaus C, Koletzko S (2001) Dumping syndrome: a common problem following Nissen fundoplication in young children. *Pediatr Surg Int* 17: 351–355.

Burgers R, De Jong TP, Benninga MA (2013) Rectal examination in children: digital versus transabdominal ultrasound. *J Urol* 190: 667–672. doi: 10.1016/j.juro.2013.02.3201.

Calis EA, Veugelers R, Sheppard JJ, Tibboel D, Evenhuis HM, Penning C (2008) Dysphagia in children with severe generalized cerebral palsy and intellectual disability. *Dev Med Child Neurol* 50: 625–630. doi: 10.1111/j.1469-8749.2008.03047.x.

Campanozzi A, Capano G, Miele E et al. (2007) Impact of malnutrition on gastrointestinal disorders and gross motor abilities in children with cerebral palsy. *Brain Dev* 29: 25–29. doi: 10.1016/j.braindev.2006.05.008.

Capriati T, Cardile S, Chiusolo F et al. (2015) Clinical management of post-pyloric enteral feeding in children. *Expert Rev Gastroenterol Hepatol* 9: 929–941. doi: 10.1586/17474124.2015.1041506.

Casas MJ, Kenny DJ, McPherson KA (1994) Swallowing/ventilation interactions during oral swallow in normal children and children with cerebral palsy. *Dysphagia* 9: 40–46.

Cheung KM, Tse PW, Ko CH, Chan YC, Laung CY, Chan KH (2001) Clinical efficacy of proton pump inhibitor therapy in neurologically impaired children with gastroesophageal reflux: prospective study. *Hong Kong Med J* 7: 356–359.

Chigira A, Omoto K, Mukai Y, Kaneko Y (1994) Lip closing pressure in disabled children: a comparison with normal children. *Dysphagia* 9: 193–198.

Clancy KJ, Hustad KC (2011) Longitudinal changes in feeding among children with cerebral palsy between the ages of 4 and 7 years. *Dev Neurorehabil* 14: 191–198. doi: 10.3109/17518423.2011.568467.

Del Giudice E, Staiano A, Capano G et al. (1999) Gastrointestinal manifestations in children with cerebral palsy. *Brain Dev* 21: 307–311.

Elawad MA, Sullivan PB (2001) Management of constipation in children with disabilities. *Dev Med Child Neurol* 43: 829–832.

Engel S, Isenmann S, Stander M, Rieger J, Bahr M, Weller M (1999) Inhibition of experimental rat glioma growth by decorin gene transfer is associated with decreased microglial infiltration. *J Neuroimmunol* 99: 13–18.

Fischer M, Adkins W, Hall L, Scaman P, Hsi S, Marlett J (1985) The effects of dietary fibre in a liquid diet on bowel function of mentally retarded individuals. *J Ment Defic Res* 29(4): 373–381.

Fried MD, Khoshoo V, Secker DJ, Gilday DL, Ash JM, Pencharz PB (1992) Decrease in gastric emptying time and episodes of regurgitation in children with spastic quadriplegia fed a whey-based formula. *J Pediatr* 120(4Pt1): 569–572. PubMed PMID: 1552396. doi: 10.1016/s0022-3476(10)80003-4.

Gisel EG (1996) Effect of oral sensorimotor treatment on measures of growth and efficiency of eating in the moderately eating-impaired child with cerebral palsy. *Dysphagia* 11: 48–58.

Griggs CA, Jones PM, Lee RE (1989) Videofluoroscopic investigation of feeding disorders of children with multiple handicap. *Dev Med Child Neurol* 31: 303–308.

Gustafsson PM, Tibbling L (1994) Gastro-oesophageal reflux and oesophageal dysfunction in children and adolescents with brain damage. *Acta Paediatrica* 83: 1081–1085.

Hirata GC, Santos RS (2012) Rehabilitation of oropharyngeal dysphagia in children with cerebral palsy: a systematic review of the speech therapy approach. *Int Arch Otorhinolaryngol* 16: 396–399. doi: 10.7162/s1809-97772012000300016.

Kawai M, Kawahara H, Hirayama S, Yoshimura N, Ida S (2004) Effect of baclofen on emesis and 24-hour esophageal pH in neurologically impaired children with gastroesophageal reflux disease. *J Pediatr Gastroent Nutr* 38: 317–323.

Kenny DJ, Casas MJ, McPherson KA (1989) Correlation of ultrasound imaging of oral swallow with ventilatory alterations in cerebral palsied and normal children: preliminary observations. *Dysphagia* 4: 112–117.

Khoshoo V, Zembo M, King A, Dhar M, Reifen R, Pencharz P (1996) Incidence of gastroesophageal reflux with whey- and casein-based formulas in infants and in children with severe neurological impairment. *J Pediatr Gastroent Nutr* 22: 48–55.

Kim S, Koh H, Lee J (2017) Gastroesophageal reflux in neurologically impaired children: what are the risk factors? *Gut Liver* 11: 232–236. doi: 10.5009/gnl16150.

King SK, Sutcliffe JR, Southwell BR, Chait PG, Hutson J (2005) The antegrade continence enema successfully treats idiopathic slow-transit constipation. *J Pediatr Surg* 40: 1935–1940. doi: 10.1016/j.jpedsurg.2005.08.011.

Kunisaki SM, Dakhoub A, Jarboe MD, Geiger JD (2011) Gastric dissociation for the treatment of congenital microgastria with paraesophageal hiatal hernia. *J Pediatr Surg* 46: e1–4. doi: 10.1016/j.jpedsurg.2011.02.048.

Lansdale N, McNiff M, Morecroft J, Kauffmann L, Morabito A (2015) Long-term and 'patient-reported' outcomes of total esophagogastric dissociation versus laparoscopic fundoplication for gastroesophageal reflux disease in the severely neurodisabled child. *J Pediatr Surg* 50: 1828–1832. doi: 10.1016/j.jpedsurg.2015.06.021.

Larnert G, Ekberg O (1995) Positioning improves the oral and pharyngeal swallowing function in children with cerebral palsy. *Acta Paediatrica* 84: 689–692.

Livingston MH, Shawyer AC, Rosenbaum PL, Jones SA, Walton JM (2015) Fundoplication and gastrostomy versus percutaneous gastrojejunostomy for gastroesophageal reflux in children with neurologic impairment: a systematic review and meta-analysis. *J Pediatr Surg* 50: 707–714. doi: 10.1016/j.jpedsurg.2015.02.020.

Miamoto CB, Ramos Jorge ML, Pereira LJ, Paiva SM, Pordeus IA, Marques LS (2010) Severity of malocclusion in patients with cerebral palsy: determinant factors. *Am J Orth Dentofac Orthoped* 138: 394.e1–5; discussion 394–395. doi: 10.1016/j.ajodo.2010.03.025.

Mirrett PL, Riski JE, Glascott J, Johnson V (1994) Videofluoroscopic assessment of dysphagia in children with severe spastic cerebral palsy. *Dysphagia* 9: 174–179.

Miyazawa R, Tomomasa T, Kaneko H, Arakawa H, Shimizu N, Morikawa A (2008) Effects of pectin liquid on gastroesophageal reflux disease in children with cerebral palsy. *BMC Gastroenterol* 8: 11. doi: 10.1186/1471-230x-8-11.

Morgan AT, Dodrill P, Ward E (2012) Interventions for oropharyngeal dysphagia in children with neurological impairment. *Cochrane Database Syst Rev* 10: Cd009456. doi: 10.1002/14651858.CD009456.pub2.

Morton RE, Bonas R, Fourie B, Minford J (1993) Videofluoroscopy in the assessment of feeding disorders of children with neurological problems. *Dev Med Child Neurol* 35: 388–395.

Neuman A, Desai B, Glass D, Diab W (2014) Superior mesenteric artery syndrome in a patient with cerebral palsy. *Case Rep Med*: 538289. doi: 10.1155/2014/538289.

Noll L, Rommel N, Davidson GP, Omari TI (2011) Pharyngeal flow interval: a novel impedance-based parameter correlating with aspiration. *Neurogastroenterol Motil* 23: 551–e206. doi: 10.1111/j.1365-2982.2010.01634.x.

O'Loughlin EV, Somerville H, Shun A et al. (2013) Antireflux surgery in children with neurological impairment: caregiver perceptions and complications. *J Pediatr Gastroent Nutr* 56: 46–50. doi: 10.1097/MPG.0b013e318267c320.

Ortega Ade O, Ciamponi AL, Mendes FM, Santos MT (2009) Assessment scale of the oral motor performance of children and adolescents with neurological damages. *J Oral Rehab* 36: 653–659. doi: 10.1111/j.1365-2842.2009.01979.x.

Otapowicz D, Sobaniec W, Okurowska-Zawada B et al. (2010) Dysphagia in children with infantile cerebral palsy. *Adv Med Sci* 55: 222–227. doi: 10.2478/v10039-010-0034-3.

Ozdemirkiran T, Secil Y, Tarlaci S, Ertekin C (2007) An EMG screening method (dysphagia limit) for evaluation of neurogenic dysphagia in childhood above 5 years old. *Int J Pediatr Otorhinolaryngol* 71: 403–407. doi: 10.1016/j.ijporl.2006.11.006.

Park ES, Park CI, Cho SR, Na SI, Cho Y (2004) Colonic transit time and constipation in children with spastic cerebral palsy. *Arch Phys Med Rehab* 85: 453–456.

Pashankar DS, Bishop WP (2001) Efficacy and optimal dose of daily polyethylene glycol 3350 for treatment of constipation and encopresis in children. *J Pediatr* 139: 428–432. doi: 10.1067/mpd.2001.117002.

Quitadamo P, Thapar N, Staiano A, Borrelli O (2016) Gastrointestinal and nutritional problems in neurologically impaired children. *Eur J Paediatr Neurol* 20: 810–815. doi: 10.1016/j.ejpn.2016.05.019.

Reilly S, Skuse D, Mathisen B, Wolke D (1995) The objective rating of oral-motor functions during feeding. *Dysphagia* 10: 177–191.

Reilly S, Skuse D, Poblete X (1996) Prevalence of feeding problems and oral motor dysfunction in children with cerebral palsy: a community survey. *J Pediatr* 129: 877–882.

Reyes AL, Cash AJ, Green SH, Booth IW (1993) Gastrooesophageal reflux in children with cerebral palsy. *Child Care Health Dev* 19: 109–118.

Reynolds J, Carroll S, Sturdivant C (2016) Fiberoptic endoscopic evaluation of swallowing: a multidisciplinary alternative for assessment of infants with dysphagia in the neonatal intensive care unit. *Adv Neonatal Care* 16: 37–43. doi: 10.1097/anc.0000000000000245.

Richards CA, Milla PJ, Andrews PL, Spitz L (2001) Retching and vomiting in neurologically impaired children after fundoplication: predictive preoperative factors. *J Pediatr Surg* 36: 1401–1404. doi: 10.1053/jpsu.2001.26384.

Rodriguez L, Flores A, Gilchrist BF, Goldstein AM (2011) Laparoscopic-assisted percutaneous endoscopic cecostomy in children with defecation disorders (with video). *Gastrointest Endosc* 73: 98–102. doi: 10.1016/j.gie.2010.09.011.

Romano C, Van Wynckel M, Hulst J et al. (2017) European Society for Paediatric Gastroenterology, Hepatology and Nutrition guidelines for the evaluation and treatment of gastrointestinal and nutritional complications in children with neurological impairment. *J Pediatr Gastroent Nutr* 65: 242–264. doi: 10.1097/mpg.0000000000001646.

Rommel N, Dejaeger E, Bellon E, Smet M, Veereman-Wauters G (2006) Videomanometry reveals clinically relevant parameters of swallowing in children. *Int J Pediatr Otorhinolaryngol* 70: 1397–1405. doi: 10.1016/j.ijporl.2006.02.005.

Sellers D, Mandy A, Pennington L, Hankins M, Morris C (2014) Development and reliability of a system to classify the eating and drinking ability of people with cerebral palsy. *Dev Med Child Neurol* 56: 245–251. doi: 10.1111/dmcn.12352.

Selley WG, Parrot LC, Lethbridge PC et al. (2000) Non-invasive technique for assessment and management planning of oral-pharyngeal dysphagia in children with cerebral palsy. *Dev Med Child Neurol* 42: 617–623.

Sullivan PB (2008) Gastrointestinal disorders in children with neurodevelopmental disabilities. *Dev Disabil Res Rev* 14: 128–136. doi: 10.1002/ddrr.18.

Takano K, Kurose M, Mitsuzawa H, Nagaya T, Himi T (2015) Clinical outcomes of tracheoesophageal diversion and laryngotracheal separation for aspiration in patients with severe motor and intellectual disability. *Acta Otolaryngol* 135: 1304–1310. doi: 10.3109/00016489.2015.1067905.

Talley NJ, Jones M, Nuyts G, Dubois D (2003) Risk factors for chronic constipation based on a general practice sample. *Am J Gastroenterol* 98: 1107–1111. doi: 10.1111/j.1572-0241.2003.07465.x.

Tambucci R, Thapar N, Saliakellis E et al. (2015) Op-24 esophageal baseline impedance in neurologically impaired children. *J Pediatr Gastroent Nutr* 61: 519–520. doi: 10.1097/01. mpg.0000472228.16916.62.

Turk H, Hauser B, Brecelj J, Vandenplas Y, Orel R (2013) Effect of proton pump inhibition on acid, weakly acid and weakly alkaline gastro-esophageal reflux in children. *World J Pediatr* 9: 36–41. doi: 10.1007/s12519-013-0405-5.

Ukleja A (2005) Dumping syndrome: pathophysiology and treatment. *Nutr Clin Pract* 20: 517–525. doi: 10.1177/0115426505020005517.

van den Engel-Hoek L, Erasmus CE, Van Hulst KC, Arvedson JC, De Groot IJ, De Swart BJ (2014) Children with central and peripheral neurologic disorders have distinguishable patterns of dysphagia on videofluoroscopic swallow study. *J Child Neurol* 29: 646–653. doi: 10.1177/0883073813501871.

Vandenplas Y, Rudolph CD, Di Lorenzo C et al. (2009) Pediatric gastroesophageal reflux clinical practice guidelines: joint recommendations of the North American Society for Pediatric Gastroenterology, Hepatology, and Nutrition (NASPGHAN) and the European Society for Pediatric Gastroenterology, Hepatology, and Nutrition (ESPGHAN). *J Pediatr Gastroent Nutr* 49: 498–547. doi: 10.1097/MPG.0b013e3181b7f563.

Vernon-Roberts A, Sullivan PB (2013) Fundoplication versus postoperative medication for gastro-oesophageal reflux in children with neurological impairment undergoing gastrostomy. *Cochrane Database Syst Rev*: Cd006151. doi: 10.1002/14651858.CD006151.pub3.

Veugelers R, Benninga MA, Calis EA et al. (2010) Prevalence and clinical presentation of constipation in children with severe generalized cerebral palsy. *Dev Med Child Neurol* 52: e216–221. doi: 10.1111/j.1469-8749.2010.03701.x.

Wales PW, Diamond IR, Dutta S et al. (2002) Fundoplication and gastrostomy versus image-guided gastrojejunal tube for enteral feeding in neurologically impaired children with gastroesophageal reflux. *J Pediatr Surg* 37: 407–412.

Yang WT, Loveday EJ, Metreweli C, Sullivan PB (1997) Ultrasound assessment of swallowing in malnourished disabled children. *Br J Radiol* 70: 992–994. doi: 10.1259/bjr.70.838.9404200.

CHAPTER 5

Consequences of Nutritional Impairment

Jessie M Hulst

INTRODUCTION

The gastrointestinal problems, oral motor dysfunction, immobility and dentition problems described in the previous chapters contribute to nutritional impairment of children with neurological impairment (NI) (Andrew et al. 2012). The term nutritional impairment used refers to undernutrition, malnutrition or poor nutritional status due to inadequate nutritional intake. Studies have shown that feeding difficulties and nutritional problems are frequent in children with NI (Stallings et al. 1993; Reilly et al. 1996; Fung et al. 2002; Andrew et al. 2012).

There is a strong relation between the grade of disability, the severity of feeding problems, nutritional intake and nutritional status in these children. Nutritional impairment can affect several physical and psychological functions leading to clinical consequences and is associated with worse outcome (Fung et al. 2002; Stevenson et al. 2006b). These consequences include undernutrition, growth failure, micronutrient deficiencies and poor bone health; they will be outlined in the following paragraphs. Figure 5.1 depicts the relationships between factors contributing to feeding difficulties, inadequate nutritional intake and its consequences in children with neurological impairment.

On the other hand there is some evidence that those children with NI with less severe motor impairments may be at increased risk of becoming overweight (Rogozinski et al.

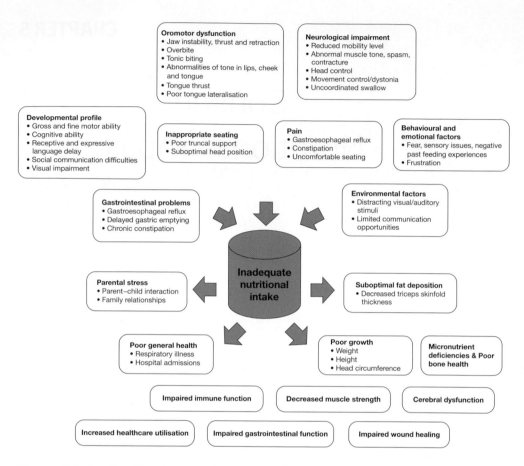

Figure 5.1 Relationships between factors contributing to feeding difficulties, inadequate nutritional intake and its consequences in children with neurological impairment. (Adapted from Andrew et al. 2012 with permission from BMJ Publishing Group Ltd.)

2007; Hurvitz et al. 2008), as are those immobile children receiving gastrostomy feeding. Gastrostomy feeding improves overall weight gain, but has been associated with excess deposition of fat (Sullivan et al. 2006). A study in the USA showed that the prevalence of obesity (based on BMI-for-age > 95th centile) in ambulatory children (GMFCS level I–III) with cerebral palsy (CP) increased from 7.7% in 1994 to 16.5% up to 2004 (Rogozinski et al. 2007). Children with a lesser degree of involvement showed the highest odds of becoming obese. In two other large cohorts of ambulatory children with CP in Korea (Park et al. 2011) and Australia (Pascoe et al. 2016), 11.2% and 7.3% of children were overweight; obesity was identified in 5.8% and 12.1%. In the Australian study, children with GMFCS level III were more likely to be overweight or obese than children with GMFCS level I (Pascoe et al. 2016).

CLINICAL CONSEQUENCES

An overview of the clinical consequences associated with nutritional impairment are shown in Table 5.1.

To examine the associations of impaired nutritional status or impaired intake of nutrients on outcome parameters, it would be necessary to compare two groups with the same condition, one with impaired nutritional status/intake and one without. In clinical practice this can be very difficult to achieve especially in children with severe neurological impairments. That is why well-performed studies are lacking. In reality, some of the consequences may also only be recognised when the nutritional status and/or nutritional intake has improved, for example the child can be more cheerful, more relaxed, less irritable and less often sick (Marchand et al. 2006).

Growth Failure: Low Weight/Impaired Height and Decreased Head Growth

The most obvious sign of poor nutritional intake is poor weight gain or loss of body weight, due to loss of fat and muscle mass. In general, the pattern of change in body composition will depend on the previous storage of fat and muscle and on sex. Depending on which definition is used for nutritional status – BMI/weight-for-age/weight-for-height/skinfold thickness – and depending on the included type of patients in terms of severity and region in the world, various prevalence rates of malnutrition are reported, most often from studies in children with CP. These rates are between 20–90% (Stallings et al. 1993; Stevenson et al. 1994; Marchand et al. 2006, 2006b; Kuperminc & Stevenson 2008; Hariprasad et al. 2017; Minocha et al. 2018).

Sustained nutritional imbalances in children can also result in impaired linear growth (stunting) and decreased head growth. Children with CP tend to be smaller and grow more slowly than typically developing children and the differences in growth increase with advancing age (Stevenson et al. 1994; Samson-Fang & Stevenson 1998). Malnutrition appears to be a major contributing cause but other factors such as endocrine dysfunction are also important (Stallings et al. 1993, 1996; Stevenson et al. 1994; Samson-Fang & Stevenson 1998).

Stunting has been described especially in children with NI and severe motor impairments (Stevenson et al. 2006b; Dabydeen et al. 2008; Hariprasad et al. 2017). It is important to realise that stunting or thinness based on BMI does not have to occur together with undernutrition/wasting as the percentage of body fat assessed by skinfold measurements or dual-energy X-ray absorptiometry can be normal or high (Finbraten et al. 2015).

Table 5.1 Consequences of impaired nutritional status and inadequate nutritional intake in children with neurological impairment (see text for references). (Reprinted from Kecskemethy & Harcke 2014 with permission from IOS Press.)

Consequence
Growth failure – undernutrition
Low weight (wasting)
Impaired linear growth (stunting)
Decreased head growth
Cerebral dysfunction
Reduced potential
Poor concentration
Reduced responsivity
Withdrawal/irritability
Worsening of epilepsy
Depression/apathy
Decreased muscle strength
Decreased respiratory muscle
Increased work of breathing
Weak cough
Impaired cardiac function
Increased circulation time
Poor healing
Micronutrient deficiencies
Low iron: associated with anaemia, fatigue, irritability, cognitive deficits, behavioural abnormalities
Low zinc: associated with anorexia, alopecia, eczema, diarrhoea, reduced growth, skin lesions, stomatitis, impaired wound healing, frequent infections
Low copper: associated with sideroblastic anaemia, reduced growth, osteoporosis, peripheral neuropathy, increased susceptibility to infections
Low folic acid: associated with megaloblastic anaemia, anorexia, behavioural changes, reduced growth
Low vitamin B12: associated with megaloblastic anaemia, muscle weakness, ataxia, spasticity, incontinence
Low vitamin D: associated with osteomalacia/penia, rickets, muscle weakness, decreased immunity, caries, hypocalcaemia, hypophosphataemia
Low carnitine: decreased muscle tone or muscle weakness, fatigue, irritability, poor feeding in infant, hypoglycaemia, cardiomyopathy
Poor bone health (demineralisation/fractures)
Impaired immune function
Increased risk of infections

(continued on next page)

Table 5.1 Consequences of impaired nutritional status and inadequate nutritional intake in children with neurological impairment (see text for references). (Reprinted from Kecskemethy & Harcke 2014 with permission from IOS Press.) (continued)

Impaired wound healing
Poor healing (especially pressure sores)
Impaired gastrointestinal function
Increased healthcare utilisation
Increase in complication rate
Increase in hospital admission and doctor's visits
Increase in length of hospital stay
Decreased level of child and family societal participation
Increased number of missed school days
Increased number of missed family activities
Decreased quality of life/general well-being

The relationship between head growth and poor nutritional intake is shown in a few interventional studies in children with neurological impairments. Additional nasogastric tube feeding improved growth and gross motor functioning compared to a group who did not receive supplements (Campanozzi et al. 2007). Another study looking into the effects of a high-energy and high-protein diet showed increased head circumference and corticospinal tract diameter in infants with perinatal brain injury when compared to infants with normal intake (Dabydeen et al. 2008).

Cerebral Function

Adequate macro- and micronutrient intake are essential for healthy brain development (Lucas et al. 1998). So, in general, learning, behaviour and cognitive functioning can be influenced by nutrition in several ways and at different periods throughout childhood. This has been shown in studies of infants with failure to thrive who were assessed in primary care and hospital clinics at childhood age (Corbett & Drewett 2004). A small-scale study (n = 20, age 5–7 years and 8–10 years) from India investigating the association between stunting and/or wasting (as a result of chronic protein-energy malnutrition) and cognitive development found that malnourished children performed poorly compared with well-nourished children on tests of attention, working memory, learning and memory, and visuospatial ability. Malnourished children, in particular those with stunting, showed a lack of age-related improvement on tests of design fluency, working memory, visual construction, learning and memory (Kar et al. 2008). A large study in children of 8 years of age, The Avon Longitudinal Study of Parents and Children in the UK, found that early growth faltering (defined as < 5th centile for weight gain in the first 8 weeks) was associated with a significantly lower total intelligence quotient by an average of –2.71 points at 8 years of age (Emond et al. 2007).

Studies looking into cerebral function in relation to nutritional status or nutrient intake in children with NI are scarce, but urgently needed (Dan 2016). As adequate macro- and micronutrient intake is needed to support brain development, nutritional inadequacy may limit the brain's capacity for remodelling and repair after injury. This issue is very relevant to children with NI since they suffer neurological injury and they often have inadequate or suboptimal nutrient intake.

A recent double blind randomised controlled trial investigating the effect of early 2-year phosphatidylcholine precursor supplementation (DHA, choline and UMP) in infants with suspected CP showed no statistically significant neurodevelopmental advantage for the treatment group as compared to the control group. There was, however, a clinically meaningful cognitive and language advantage found in the treatment group (Andrew et al. 2015, 2018).

Clinically meaningful changes in the outcome of children with NI such as less irritability, improved responsiveness, better concentration and less apathy are also frequently reported by parents but not adequately studied.

Decreased Muscle Strength

Protein and energy malnutrition can lead to reduced lean body mass which is associated with decreased muscle strength. In healthy individuals, muscle function, as assessed by grip strength, is directly proportional to indices of body muscle mass. It has been suggested that impaired muscle function during low energy intake and malnutrition could be, apart from reduced muscle mass, related to several factors, for example alterations in numbers of muscle fibres, changes in activities of muscle enzymes, defects in calcium channels or sodium-potassium ATPase pumps (Stratton et al. 2003).

Several studies in adults with various diseases have shown associations between loss of muscle mass and outcome parameters such as postoperative complications after gastrointestinal surgery and mortality (Stratton et al. 2003).

In general, malnutrition can also result in loss of cardiac muscle which can result in decreased cardiac output, bradycardia, hypotension and peripheral circulation failure; the last sign is frequently seen in children with NI in clinical practice.

Moreover, malnutrition and protein depletion can adversely affect respiratory muscle structure and function, resulting in reduced muscle mass of the diaphragm and reduced respiratory muscle strength. Impaired respiratory function and muscle strength will weaken the cough and impair airway clearance, which may predispose to and delay recovery form chest infections. Although specific studies in children with NI about the association between nutritional status, muscle strength and adverse events are lacking, these associations are highly relevant in this population as they frequently experience chest infections (Boel et al. 2018). One study in a small group of children with spastic quadriplegic CP that assessed the health status before, at and 6 months after gastrostomy tube placement showed an improvement in nutritional status over time and in 50% of children a decrease in the number of chest infections requiring antibiotics was seen after 6 months (Vernon-Roberts et al. 2010).

Micronutrient Deficiencies

Poor overall nutritional intake can lead to lower micronutrient intake, which predisposes children with NI to develop micronutrient deficiencies. In general, micronutrients are important for many metabolic pathways in the body and generalised or specific micronutrient deficiencies may have multiple consequences (Table 5.1). These consequences may be difficult to distinguish from the general neurological impairment of NI children as they may affect cognition, behaviour, social interaction and developmental outcomes.

Few studies have evaluated the micronutrient status of children with NI and the implications of various deficiencies on health outcome (Sanchez-Lastres et al. 2003; Hillesund et al. 2007; Tomoum et al. 2010; Kalra et al. 2015; Takeda et al. 2015). These studies show that deficiencies for iron, zinc, copper, vitamin D, carnitine, folic acid and vitamin B12 are common with percentages ranging between 10% and 55%. Factors associated with low levels were found to be vitamin C intake (iron), use of antiepileptic drugs (carnitine, vitamin B12, folic acid, calcium and phosphorus), and reduced exposure to sunlight (vitamin D).

Tube feeding and the use of nutritional supplements were associated with higher concentrations of micronutrients in blood and serum (Hillesund et al. 2007). On the other hand it is also known that deficiencies in micronutrients can still occur when children with NI are exclusively tube fed with a standard formula (Piccoli et al. 2002). Children with NI may require less energy in order to avoid becoming overweight and, as a consequence of a reduced energy intake, their micronutrient intake can be less than daily requirements. Essential fatty acid (FA) deficiency may also be related to suboptimal energy intake as was shown in a study where children with NI were found to have lower levels of docosahexaenoic acid, linoleic acid and total n-6FA in comparison with a healthy reference group (Hals et al. 2000).

The monitoring of micronutrient status in NI children may have a substantial and measurable impact on their nutritional adequacy, hospital costs and future outcomes. In their recent guidelines for the evaluation and treatment of nutritional complications in children with neurological impairment, The European Society for Paediatric Gastroenterology Hepatology and Nutrition (ESPGHAN) recommends the assessment of micronutrient status (e.g. vitamin D, iron, calcium, phosphorus) as part of nutritional assessment and that micronutrients should be checked annually (Romano et al. 2017).

ESPGHAN also recommends use of the dietary reference intake for micronutrients in typically developing children to estimate the appropriate micronutrient intake for NI children (Romano et al. 2017).

Iron

Iron deficiency is a common problem in children with NI (Sullivan et al. 2002; Papadopoulos et al. 2008) and is related to insufficient intake and inadequate iron absorption. Children with NI on a liquid diet were found to have higher rates of anaemia and iron deficiency compared to children on a normal diet. Prepared liquid diets, although including various types of food, may consist of foods that are a poor source of iron (milk, cheese, cream, yoghurt, rice) or that inhibit iron absorption (vegetables, grains, pulses, cereals) (Papadopoulos et al. 2008).

Since iron deficiency is associated with anaemia, cognitive deficits and behavioural abnormalities, it is important to monitor and supplement when needed. The recommended daily intake of iron is 10mg/day in children (7–10 years), 12mg/day in adolescent males (15–19 years) and 15mg/day in adolescent females (15–19 years). In the treatment of iron deficiency in children with NI it is reasonable to provide iron supplementation as the first diagnostic and therapeutic measure in such patients.

Vitamin D

Decreased 25-hydroxy vitamin D is a major deficiency noted and besides inadequate food intake, inadequate exposure to sunlight and the use of anticonvulsants can be additional risk factors in this group of children. Anticonvulsants can increase the activity of cytochrome P450 mixed function oxidase enzyme, which results in the conversion of vitamin D to an inactive metabolite.

Poor Bone Health

Low bone mineralisation (osteopenia and osteoporosis) is a severe and frequently encountered problem in children with NI and is associated with significant fracture risk. There are multiple factors that can contribute to poor bone health which can all be present in children with NI: vitamin D deficiency, poor intake of calcium and phosphorous, limited ambulation (GMFCS level IV and V), feeding difficulties, low weight-for-age, previous fracture, anticonvulsant use and lower fat mass (Duncan et al. 1999; Henderson et al. 2002; Stevenson et al. 2006a; Mergler et al. 2009; Bianchi et al. 2014). Rickets is infrequently seen in this population because it is a disease of growing children and many children with CP are growing poorly or not at all. This issue is covered in detail in Chapter 8.

Impaired Immune Function and Increased Infection

Protein-energy malnutrition and micronutrient deficiencies can negatively influence the haematopoietic and lymphoid organs and compromise both innate and adaptive immune functions. These changes are associated with impaired ability to prevent, fight and recover from various types of infections. Most of the knowledge about the impact of malnutrition on host defence comes from animal studies and studies in children in developing countries (Ibrahim et al. 2017).

Skin, respiratory and gastrointestinal mucosal barrier integrity can be impaired in children with malnutrition. Children with neurological impairment are prone to respiratory infections (Millman et al. 2016) because of a combination of factors such as decline in lung function, respiratory muscle weakness or atrophy, increased bacterial colonisation of airways and decreased resistance to infection (Boel et al. 2018). Poor nutritional status and decreased nutritional intake may be an important additional risk affecting the different factors.

Micronutrient deficiencies, such as deficiencies of iron, zinc, selenium and vitamins A/C/D, can also have a profound effect on immune function and host defence (Ibrahim et al. 2017). Because children with NI frequently show inadequate micronutrient status, this is highly relevant to this group, and may further contribute to the increased susceptibility to infections and their severity.

Impaired Wound Healing

Nutrition plays an important role in the complex process of wound healing and the development of wounds such as pressure ulcers. Among other factors – for example local factors, presence of chronic disease and age – nutritional status and recent nutritional intake seem to be especially important (Clark et al. 2000). Several studies showed impaired or prolonged wound healing in malnourished patients when compared to patients with normal nutritional status.

Malnutrition goes together with reduced nutrient availability for metabolism, maintenance and repair; losses of fat; physical weakness; decreases in skin resistance; edema; and decreased motility, which are associated with the risk of pressure ulcer development. Specific micronutrient deficiencies, such as vitamin A, vitamin C, vitamin E and zinc, may also play a role in this increased risk. This has been shown by a number of studies, not specifically in individuals with NI. In children with NI several risk factors may be present besides poor nutritional status and nutritional intake, such as less activity (wheelchair bound, bed bound), incontinence (moisture), loss of sensations (reduced pain sensation that would normally cause an immobile individual to change position), contractures and spasticity (repeated exposure of tissues to pressure through flexion of a joint).

A retrospective study among 79 children with CP who underwent hip surgeries concluded that risk factors for complications were non-ambulant status and on top of this the presence of gastrostomy feeding, indicating the role of nutritional status. Gross motor function correlated well with the risk of complications after osteotomies (Stasikelis et al. 1999).

Another recent study in patients undergoing posterior spine fusion for neuromuscular scoliosis consecutive to CP (n = 66) or muscular dystrophy (n = 30) showed a high rate of early complications especially in the CP group (59%) and especially infectious complications (32%). Infectious complications included 16 wound infections (16.7%) and associations with a lower body weight and poor nutritional status were found (Pesenti et al. 2016).

Impaired Intestinal Function

Adequate nutrition is important for preserving gut structure and function, including digestion and absorption of nutrients and providing the gut barrier. Changes in gastrointestinal structure and function can be seen especially when luminal nutrition is lacking (Stratton et al. 2003). These effects may not be apparent in situations with chronic energy restriction with preserved (minimal) enteral nutrition even though body weight may be dramatically decreased. Few human studies have been performed about the effects of acute and chronic food deprivation on the gastrointestinal tract (absorption, intestinal permeability and transit time), and no studies are available in children with NI. The most evident effect of acute starvation is a reduction of small bowel absorptive surface area due to villous blunting, leading to impaired absorption of monosaccharide and disaccharide that can contribute to diarrhoea (Kvissberg et al. 2016). On the other hand, compensatory mechanisms leading to maximisation of nutrient absorption also come into play. Therefore the clinical significance of changes in gut structure and function in case of malnutrition remain unclear. It is known however that effects of malnutrition on the gut can be more pronounced in the presence of acute illness.

Specific micronutrient deficiencies may also have an effect on intestinal morphology, for example vitamin B2.

It is well known that NI can affect the gastrointestinal system, most notably the oral motor function and motility. The association between nutritional status and gastrointestinal problems in NI children is not well studied. A small uncontrolled study among 21 children with CP and severe intellectual disability looked at the relationship between nutritional status and gastrointestinal problems (gastroesophageal reflux disease [GERD] and/or chronic constipation), and evaluated the role of nutrition on their gross motor abilities (Campanozzi et al. 2007). Nutritional rehabilitation (increase of daily calories by 20%) of malnourished children took place and children with GERD received additional proton pump inhibitor treatment. While the nutritional status improved, the majority of patients had persistent GERD after 6 months of combined treatment. Improved nutritional status, particularly fat free mass gain, appeared to have a positive impact on motor function in children with CP.

Increased Healthcare Utilisation

In general, malnutrition in children has been shown to be associated with an increased length of hospital stay in a number of studies (Joosten et al. 2010; Hecht et al. 2015). This increase in use of healthcare resources is likely to increase the cost of care of malnourished children. A large retrospective analysis of over 6 million hospitalised children aged < 17 years in the USA found that length of hospital stay among children with a coded diagnosis of malnutrition was significantly longer than those without. In addition, they found that discharge home with care was 3.5 times more common among malnourished patients (10.9% vs 3.1%, p < 0.001) (Abdelhadi et al. 2016). In this study hospitalisation costs were US$55 255 for children with a malnutrition diagnosis vs US$17 309 without. The higher requirement of post-discharge home care further suggests higher costs in the community as well.

The impact of poor growth and nutrition on health outcomes in children with moderate to severe CP were investigated in few studies. The children with the poorest overall growth (low arm fat and arm muscle area) had more days of health service utilisation (i.e. doctors' visits, hospitalisations) compared with those children who had the best overall growth (Samson-Fang et al. 2002). This study was the first to document a link between nutritional status, as defined by anthropometry and healthcare utilisation.

In a large multicentre study among 273 children with moderate and severe CP (GMFCS II–IV–V) healthcare use (days in bed, days in hospital and visits to doctor or emergency department) and social participation (days missed of school or of usual activities for child and family) over the preceding 4 weeks were measured by questionnaire. The results showed that children with the best growth had fewest days of healthcare use and fewest days of social participation missed, whereas the children with the worst growth had the most days of healthcare use and most days of participation missed (Stevenson et al. 2006b).

Level of Child and Family Societal Participation

The impact of poor growth and nutrition on levels of participation in children with moderate to severe CP was also incorporated in the study of Samson-Fang and colleagues (Samson-Fang et al. 2002). Low arm fat and arm muscle area were associated with decreased global health scores, and child and family societal participation. Children with poorest overall growth had lower levels of participation compared with those children who had the best overall growth.

Data in children with CP from The North American Growth in Cerebral Palsy Project showed that low fat stores were associated with lower global health scores, less child and family participation and increased use of health care (Liptak et al. 2001).

Quality of Life

Children with NI have a reduced health-related quality of life (QoL) and the degree is related to the severity of their NI (Samson-Fang et al. 2002; Vargus-Adams 2005). The presence and severity of malnutrition and of feeding problems both have an impact on QoL. Studies directly addressing the relationship between nutritional status, nutritional problems and QoL in children with NI are lacking, but there are some studies looking into QoL after initiating tube feeding with subsequent improvement in nutritional status. A prospective longitudinal study addressing QoL before and after gastrostomy or gastrojejunal tube insertion showed a mean increase in weight for age z-score from –2.8 at baseline to –1.8 at 12 months, with no increase in mean parental-rated QoL and health-related QoL scores in the same period. However, parents felt that the tube had a positive impact on their child's health, particularly with regards to feeding and administration of medications (Mahant et al. 2009).

Indirectly, it has also been shown that the quality of life of caregivers of children with CP can significantly be improved after insertion of a gastrostomy feeding tube in the child in their care, in terms of significant reduction in feeding times, increased ease of drug administration and reduced concern about the child's nutritional status (Sullivan et al. 2004).

On the other hand, being overweight or obese, which is becoming more prevalent in ambulatory children with NI (Pascoe et al. 2016), can also be an important topic in relation to QoL. For children with NI who may already have difficulties with body image and may experience prejudice and discrimination, the combination of being overweight or obese with physical disability can impact QoL to a greater degree than in children who are obese but do not have a physical disability (Rimmer et al. 2011). Increased body mass in conjunction with increasing musculoskeletal impairments may result in progressive loss of function and mobility when compared with peers without a disability (Park et al. 2011).

Mortality

Although high-quality studies specifically addressing children with NI are lacking and data demonstrating that malnutrition has an adverse impact on morbidity and mortality in paediatrics is limited, it is clear from extrapolation of studies in adults and from studies in children in developing countries that malnutrition is associated with a greater risk (Moy et al. 1990; Stratton et al. 2003). A small recent study about risk factors for mortality in children with CP in Indonesia reported on nutritional status but could not relate it to increased mortality risk (Prastiya et al. 2018). A 1-year follow-up study in 81 children and adolescents with CP in Chile did not find an increased mortality in children at high nutritional risk, but both nutritional risk and mortality were found to be significantly higher in gastrostomy-fed children (RR 2,98 CI 95%: 1.32–6.75 combining both variables) (Figueroa et al. 2017). A possible reason for this is that gastrostomy tube feeding is in itself an indicator of severity of impairment and therefore of an increased risk of mortality.

SUMMARY

Children with NI frequently have nutritional impairment due to inadequate nutritional intake and this has enormous impact on overall health and QoL. There is a strong relation between the grade of general motor function and cognitive ability, the severity of feeding problems, nutritional intake and nutritional status in these children. Nutritional assessment and support should be an integral part of the care of children with NI aiming at early identification of children at risk of nutrition-related comorbidities. To ensure success of interventions, a multidisciplinary team should perform close monitoring of nutritional status.

Case Study

An 18-year-old boy with severe intellectual and motoric disability because of a chromosomal disorder, known with tetraplegic spasticity and GMCFS level IV, was admitted to undergo several orthopaedic surgical corrections in one session. He had been on the waiting list for more than 18 months and was followed by the rehabilitation physician. His preoperative anaesthetic screening took place 2 days before the planned surgery and a weight of 38kg and height of 160cm were obtained. His nutritional status parameters were automatically calculated in the digital patient system and were: WFA –5.1SD, WFH –2.2SD and HFA –3.9SD based on national reference for healthy children, indicating undernutrition. He was used to eating orally and parents told that he enjoyed that.

All surgical interventions went well, but took a total of 11 hours. Postoperatively he developed several problems including respiratory failure because of aspiration pneumonia necessitating non-invasive ventilation at the paediatric intensive care unit and an extended length of hospital stay. In addition he developed a pressure sore at the left knee and severe nutritional problems necessitating nasojejunal tube feeding. After one month, he was discharged home with a weight of 33.7kg (WFA –6.08SD, BMI –7.1SD based on healthy population reference) with additional measures including sputum drainage system and tube feeding.

Already after one day he was re-admitted to the paediatric ward because of respiratory problems with aspiration of enteral formula. He was very tired, not able to sit for more than

15 minutes and showed signs of skin pressure at his spine. As he was not able to tolerate enteral nutrition, he was started on parenteral nutrition to try to let him gain some weight and recover. Because of increasing respiratory problems with incidents with low saturation, because of inability to clear sputum and swallowing difficulties, he was transported to paediatric intensive care again for non-invasive ventilatory support. After some clinical improvement, a barium contrast swallowing study was performed which showed an unsafe swallowing with aspiration. After careful discussion with parents and the treatment team, it was decided to give him a jejunostomy in order to try to feed him enterally as placement of nasal gastrojejunal tubes were not successful. In the days after the jejunostomy placement he developed a pneumonia again and became respiratory insufficient. After some days without improvement, it was decided to continue with palliative comfort care (no intubation) because of the total deterioration of his condition. Six weeks after the initial admission for orthopaedic surgery he sadly passed away.

- *This clinical case gives an example of how a poor nutritional status can play a role in the development of complications after surgery. A multidisciplinary assessment (surgeon, paediatrician, dietician and speech therapist/occupational therapist) in the preoperative period could have given insight about nutritional status and its contributing factors and may have led to a (nutritional) intervention in order to try to improve nutritional status before major surgery. Although it is difficult to actually tell and considering other relevant aspects in a neurologically impaired child, this may have led to a better outcome.*

REFERENCES

Abdelhadi RA, Bouma S, Bairdain S et al. (2016) Characteristics of hospitalized children with a diagnosis of malnutrition: United States, 2010. *JPEN J Parenter Enteral Nutr* 40: 623–635.

Andrew MJ, Parr JR, Sullivan PB (2012) Feeding difficulties in children with cerebral palsy. *Arch Dis Child-Ed Pract* 97: 222–229.

Andrew MJ, Parr JR, Montague-Johnson C et al. (2015) Optimising nutrition to improve growth and reduce neurodisabilities in neonates at risk of neurological impairment, and children with suspected or confirmed cerebral palsy. *BMC Pediatr* 15: 22.

Andrew MJ, Parr JR, Montague-Johnson C et al. (2018) Nutritional intervention and neurodevelopmental outcome in infants with suspected cerebral palsy: the Dolphin infant double-blind randomized controlled trial. *Dev Med Child Neurol* 60: 906–913.

Bianchi ML, Leonard MB, Bechtold S et al. (2014) Bone health in children and adolescents with chronic diseases that may affect the skeleton: the 2013 ISCD Pediatric Official Positions. *J Clin Densitom* 17: 281–294.

Boel L, Pernet K, Toussaint M et al. (2018) Respiratory morbidity in children with cerebral palsy: an overview. *Dev Med Child Neurol* 61(6): 646–653.

Campanozzi A, Capano G, Miele E et al. (2007) Impact of malnutrition on gastrointestinal disorders and gross motor abilities in children with cerebral palsy. *Brain Dev* 29: 25–29.

Clark MA, Plank LD, Hill GL (2000) Wound healing associated with severe surgical illness. *World J Surg* 24: 648–654.

Corbett SS, Drewett RF (2004) To what extent is failure to thrive in infancy associated with poorer cognitive development? A review and meta-analysis. *J Child Psychol Psychiatry* 45: 641–654.

Dabydeen L, Thomas JE, Aston TJ, Hartley H, Sinha SK, Eyre JA (2008) High-energy and -protein diet increases brain and corticospinal tract growth in term and preterm infants after perinatal brain injury. *Pediatrics* 121: 148–156.

Dan B (2016) Nutrition, brain function, and plasticity in cerebral palsy. *Dev Med Child Neurol* 58: 890.

Duncan B, Barton LL, Lloyd J, Marks-Katz M (1999) Dietary considerations in osteopenia in tube-fed nonambulatory children with cerebral palsy. *Clin Pediatr (Phila)* 38: 133–137.

Emond AM, Blair PS, Emmett PM, Drewett RF (2007) Weight faltering in infancy and IQ levels at 8 years in the Avon Longitudinal Study of Parents and Children. *Pediatrics* 120: e1051–1058.

Figueroa MJ, Rojas C, Barja S (2017) Morbimortality associated to nutritional status and feeding path in children with cerebral palsy. *Rev Chil Pediatr* 88: 478–486.

Finbraten AK, Martins C, Andersen GL et al. (2015) Assessment of body composition in children with cerebral palsy: a cross-sectional study in Norway. *Dev Med Child Neurol* 57: 858–864.

Fung EB, Samson-Fang L, Stallings VA et al. (2002) Feeding dysfunction is associated with poor growth and health status in children with cerebral palsy. *J Am Diet Assoc* 102: 361–373.

Hals J, Bjerve KS, Nilsen H, Svalastog AG, Ek J (2000) Essential fatty acids in the nutrition of severely neurologically disabled children. *Br J Nutr* 83: 219–225.

Hariprasad PG, Elizabeth KE, Valamparampil MJ, Kalpana D, Anish TS (2017) Multiple nutritional deficiencies in cerebral palsy compounding physical and functional impairments. *Indian J Palliat Care* 23: 387–392.

Hecht C, Weber M, Grote V et al. (2015) Disease associated malnutrition correlates with length of hospital stay in children. *Clin Nutr* 34: 53–59.

Henderson RC, Lark RK, Gurka MJ et al. (2002) Bone density and metabolism in children and adolescents with moderate to severe cerebral palsy. *Pediatrics* 110: e5.

Hillesund E, Skranes J, Trygg KU, Bohmer T (2007) Micronutrient status in children with cerebral palsy. *Acta Paediatrica* 96: 1195–1198.

Hurvitz EA, Green LB, Hornyak JE, Khurana SR, Koch LG (2008) Body mass index measures in children with cerebral palsy related to gross motor function classification: a clinic-based study. *Am J Phys Med Rehabil* 87: 395–403.

Ibrahim MK, Zambruni M, Melby CL, Melby PC (2017) Impact of childhood malnutrition on host defense and infection. *Clin Microbiol Rev* 30: 919–971.

Joosten KF, Zwart H, Hop WC, Hulst JM (2010) National malnutrition screening days in hospitalised children in The Netherlands. *Arch Dis Child* 95: 141–145.

Kalra S, Aggarwal A, Chillar N, Faridi MM (2015) Comparison of micronutrient levels in children with cerebral palsy and neurologically normal controls. *Indian J Pediatr* 82: 140–144.

Kar BR, Rao SL, Chandramouli BA (2008) Cognitive development in children with chronic protein energy malnutrition. *Behav Brain Funct* 4: 31.

Kecskemethy HH, Harcke HT (2014) Assessment of bone health in children with disabilities. *J Rehabil Med* 7: 111–124.

Kuperminc MN, Stevenson RD (2008) Growth and nutrition disorders in children with cerebral palsy. *Dev Disabil Res Rev* 14: 137–146.

Kvissberg MA, Dalvi PS, Kerac M et al. (2016) Carbohydrate malabsorption in acutely malnourished children and infants: a systematic review. *Nutr Rev* 74: 48–58.

Liptak GS, O'Donnell M, Conaway M et al. (2001) Health status of children with moderate to severe cerebral palsy. *Dev Med Child Neurol* 43: 364–370.

Lucas A, Morley R, Cole TJ (1998) Randomised trial of early diet in preterm babies and later intelligence quotient. *BMJ* 317: 1481–1487.

Mahant S, Friedman JN, Connolly B, Goia C, MacArthur C (2009) Tube feeding and quality of life in children with severe neurological impairment. *Arch Dis Child* 94: 668–673.

Marchand V, Motil KJ, Nutrition NCO (2006) Nutrition support for neurologically impaired children: a clinical report of the North American Society for Pediatric Gastroenterology, Hepatology, and Nutrition. *J Pediatr Gastroent Nutr* 43: 123–135.

Mergler S, Evenhuis HM, Boot AM et al. (2009) Epidemiology of low bone mineral density and fractures in children with severe cerebral palsy: a systematic review. *Dev Med Child Neurol* 51: 773–778.

Millman AJ, Finelli L, Bramley AM et al. (2016) Community-acquired pneumonia hospitalization among children with neurologic disorders. *J Pediatr* 173: 188–195-e4.

Minocha P, Sitaraman S, Choudhary A, Yadav R (2018) Subjective global nutritional assessment: a reliable screening tool for nutritional assessment in cerebral palsy children. *Indian J Pediatr* 85: 15–19.

Moy R, Smallman S, Booth I (1990) Malnutrition in a UK children's hospital. *J Hum Nutr Diet* 3: 93–100.

Papadopoulos A, Ntaios G, Kaiafa G et al. (2008) Increased incidence of iron deficiency anemia secondary to inadequate iron intake in institutionalized, young patients with cerebral palsy. *Int J Hematol* 88: 495–497.

Park ES, Chang WH, Park JH, Yoo JK, Kim SM, Rha DW (2011) Childhood obesity in ambulatory children and adolescents with spastic cerebral palsy in Korea. *Neuropediatrics* 42: 60–66.

Pascoe J, Thomason P, Graham HK, Reddihough D, Sabin MA (2016) Body mass index in ambulatory children with cerebral palsy: A cohort study. *J Paediatr Child Health* 52: 417–421.

Pesenti S, Blondel B, Peltier E et al. (2016) Experience in perioperative management of patients undergoing posterior spine fusion for neuromuscular scoliosis. *Biomed Res Int* 3053056.

Piccoli R, Gelio S, Fratucello A, Valletta E (2002) Risk of low micronutrient intake in neurologically disabled children artificially fed. *J Pediatr Gastroent Nutr* 35: 583–584.

Prastiya IG, Risky VP, Mira I, Retno AS, Darto S, Erny P (2018) Risk factor of mortality in Indonesian children with cerebral palsy. *J Med Invest* 65: 18–20.

Reilly S, Skuse D, Poblete X (1996) Prevalence of feeding problems and oral motor dysfunction in children with cerebral palsy: a community survey. *J Pediatr* 129: 877–882.

Rimmer JH, Yamaki K, Davis BM, Wang E, Vogel LC (2011) Obesity and overweight prevalence among adolescents with disabilities. *Prev Chronic Dis* 8: A41.

Rogozinski BM, Davids JR, Davis RB et al. (2007) Prevalence of obesity in ambulatory children with cerebral palsy. *J Bone Joint Surg Am* 89: 2421–2426.

Romano C, Van Wynckel M, Hulst J et al. (2017) European Society for Paediatric Gastroenterology, Hepatology and Nutrition guidelines for the evaluation and treatment of gastrointestinal and nutritional complications in children with neurological impairment. *J Pediatr Gastroent Nutr* 65: 242–264.

Samson-Fang L, Stevenson RD (1998) Linear growth velocity in children with cerebral palsy. *Dev Med Child Neurol* 40: 689–692.

Samson-Fang L, Fung E, Stallings VA et al. (2002) Relationship of nutritional status to health and societal participation in children with cerebral palsy. *J Pediatr* 141: 637–643.

Sanchez-Lastres J, Eiris-Punal J, Otero-Cepeda JL, Pavon-Belinchon P, Castro-Gago M (2003) Nutritional status of mentally retarded children in northwest spain: II. Biochemical indicators. *Acta Paediatrica* 92: 928–934.

Stallings VA, Charney EB, Davies JC, Cronk CE (1993) Nutritional status and growth of children with diplegic or hemiplegic cerebral palsy. *Dev Med Child Neurol* 35: 997–1006.

Stallings VA, Zemel BS, Davies JC, Cronk CE, Charney EB (1996) Energy expenditure of children and adolescents with severe disabilities: a cerebral palsy model. *Am J Clin Nutr* 64: 627–634.

Stasikelis PJ, Lee DD, Sullivan CM (1999) Complications of osteotomies in severe cerebral palsy. *J Pediatr Orthop* 19: 207–210.

Stevenson RD, Hayes RP, Cater LV, Blackman JA (1994) Clinical correlates of linear growth in children with cerebral palsy. *Dev Med Child Neurol* 36: 135–142.

Stevenson RD, Conaway M, Barrington JW, Cuthill SL, Worley G, Henderson RC (2006a) Fracture rate in children with cerebral palsy. *Pediatr Rehabil* 9: 396–403.

Stevenson RD, Conaway M, Chumlea WC et al. (2006b) Growth and health in children with moderate-to-severe cerebral palsy. *Pediatrics* 118: 1010–1018.

Stratton RJ, Green CJ, Elia M (2003) Consequences of disease-related malnutrition. In: *Disease-related Malnutrition: An Evidence-based Approach to Treatment*, 1st edn. Wallingford: CABI Publishing, pp. 116–118; 120–121; 143–152.

Sullivan PB, Juszczak E, Lambert BR, Rose M, Ford-Adams ME, Johnson A (2002) Impact of feeding problems on nutritional intake and growth: Oxford Feeding Study II. *Dev Med Child Neurol* 44: 461–467.

Sullivan PB, Juszczak E, Bachlet AM et al. (2004) Impact of gastrostomy tube feeding on the quality of life of carers of children with cerebral palsy. *Dev Med Child Neurol* 46: 796–800.

Sullivan PB, Alder N, Bachlet AM et al. (2006) Gastrostomy feeding in cerebral palsy: too much of a good thing? *Dev Med Child Neurol* 48: 877–882.

Takeda Y, Kubota M, Sato H et al. (2015) Carnitine in severely disabled patients: relation to anthropometric, biochemical variables, and nutritional intake. *Brain Dev* 37: 94–100.

Tomoum HY, Badawy NB, Hassan HE, Alian KM (2010) Anthropometry and body composition analysis in children with cerebral palsy. *Clin Nutr* 29: 477–481.

Vargus-Adams J (2005) Health-related quality of life in childhood cerebral palsy. *Arch Phys Med Rehabil* 86: 940–945.

Vernon-Roberts A, Wells J, Grant H et al. (2010) Gastrostomy feeding in cerebral palsy: enough and no more. *Dev Med Child Neurol* 52: 1099–1105.

CHAPTER 6

Assessment of Nutritional State: Growth, Anthropometry and Body Composition

Jane Hardy and Hayley Kuter

INTRODUCTION

Understanding the nutritional state of children with neurological impairment presents a challenge. The definition of neurodisability according to a Delphi survey conducted in the UK is a group of congenital or acquired long term conditions that are attributed to impairment of the brain or neuromuscular system and create functional limitations. A specific diagnosis may not be identified. Conditions may vary over time, occur alone or in a combination, and include a broad range of severity and complexity. The impact may include difficulties with movement, cognition, hearing and vision, communication, emotion, and behaviour (Morris et al. 2013). Using this definition allows an appreciation of the complexity of assessing the nutritional state in children with a variety of different diagnoses and needs.

Identification and treatment of poor nutrition is crucial. Steps need to be taken to recognise and avoid both under- and over-nutrition. Weight and height – as frequently used in neurotypical children – may not fully explain the nutritional state in children with neurodisability. However, there are other anthropometric methods which can be used. As we explain below, no one measure provides a complete description of nutritional state.

ANTHROPOMETRIC MEASURES

Technique and Equipment

Anthropometric assessment rests on the ability to characterise consistently and with confidence. It can be dangerously misleading to assume that simple measures are exempt from errors – unsuitable equipment, inaccurate calibration, lack of standardised techniques and poor documentation can have significant consequences (Wootton et al. 2014).

There are no internationally agreed quality standards for the measurement of stature, weight and body composition in either typically developing children or those with neurological impairment (Wootton et al. 2014). Several authorities provide differing guidelines on measurement techniques: WHO Child Growth Standards, Child Growth Foundation (UK) and the International Society for the Advancement of Kinanthropometry (de Onis et al. 2004; Stewart et al. 2011). It is crucial that interpretation of growth using reference standards follows the same protocol for measurement (de Onis et al. 2004). There is a need for a harmonised agreement on the anthropometric measurement of children.

Accurate and reliable anthropometric measurements can be established by:

- Ensuring that measuring instruments are appropriate, regularly serviced and calibrated against external reference materials

- The use of standardised operating procedures

- The use of formalised training and demonstrable competencies including acceptable technical error of measurement (TEM)

- Ensuring that reporting systems are in place to legibly record measurements

It is good practice to take all measurements twice and the average taken. See Table 6.1 for recommendations on repeat measurements.

Serial measurements taken over time provide the opportunity to assess growth velocity and can detect or assuage concerns. The frequency of measurements should be determined individually, and depend on risk factors and level of concern. Guidelines suggest that neurologically impaired infants should have their growth assessed every 1–3 months, and older children should have anthropometry measured at least every 6 months (Romano et al. 2017).

For children with cerebral palsy (CP) the Gross Motor Function Classification System (GMFCS) categorises children according to functional abilities including their mobility status. This is a well-defined group and much research has focused on children with CP.

Table 6.1 Considerations for anthropometric measurements

Measure	Equipment required	Comments on technique	Repeat measurements/ frequency
Weight	Digital scales for standers. Wheelchair, sitting or hoist scales for non-standers. Measures to a precision of 0.1kg (100g). Allows 'tared' weighing (scales can be reset to zero).	Children under 2 years should be naked. Minimal clothing for older children. For small children unwilling to be weighed on their own, an adult should stand on the scale, scales tared and child placed in adult's arms.	Take two weights and record the mean. If two weights differ by more than 100g, take a third measurement and median.
Height/Length	Measuring board for supine length in infants under 2 years. Stadiometer, mounted wall ruler or the Leicester height meter for standers. Non-standers – *see below*. Segmental measurements (knee height or tibial length): calipers or segmometer, tape measure.	Scoliosis, joint contractures, spasticity, dystonia and agitation will interfere with optimal positioning. Protocols for measurement should include positioning of the individual (Frankfort plane, whether to 'stretch' with an inhalation) and position of measurers. Diurnal variation in height (by up to 1%) can occur meaning that repeat measures should be taken at the same time of day if possible (Reilly et al. 1984). The 'stretch' method reduces the effect of this.	Two measurements should be taken and averaged.
Skinfolds	Calipers – calibrated to 0.2mm – exert constant pressure of 10g/mm²	Reading taken 2 seconds after caliper is applied. Skinfolds may be easier to perform in non-standers than standers.	Two measures taken, at least 2 minutes apart, and averaged. A third measurement should be taken if the difference is more than 0.2mm apart, and the median recorded.

(continued on next page)

Table 6.1 Considerations for anthropometric measurements (continued)

Measure	Equipment required	Comments on technique	Repeat measurements/ frequency
Body circumferences	Tape measure – not stretchable Segmometer or calipers to measure mid-point of upper arm	MUAC to be measured at the mid-point[a] of the upper arm Waist circumference includes: (1) True waist circumference: mid-point between 10th rib and the iliac crest; (2) Umbilical waist circumference: at the level of the umbilicus	Two measurements should be taken and averaged If two measurements differ by more than 0.2cm then a third measurement should be taken and the median recorded
Bioelectrical impedance analysis (BIA)	Weight and height must be measured prior to BIA BIA instruments use either leg-to-leg or arm-to-leg technique	Because of differences in hydration, ensure measurements are made when the child is well and repeat measurements taken at the same time of day	Consider taking two measurements and calculating the mean
Dual-energy X-ray absorptiometry (DXA)	Specialist equipment required	Ionising radiation is used; but doses are low	

[a] Location of mid-point of upper arm will depend on the method chosen (e.g. Tanner & Whitehouse 1975; Stewart et al. 2011).

However, children with neurodisability are a heterogeneous group and we have found that the reliability of anthropometric measurements differs between children who can stand unassisted ('standers') and those who cannot stand unassisted ('non-standers') (Hardy et al. 2018).

Weight

Weight has been used in a number of different ways to assess nutritional status in neurologically impaired children. Weight for age, weight for height and body mass index (BMI) all employ the simple technique of weighing the child. Weight is the sum of fat, muscle, bone, body organs and fluids. A gain or loss of weight does not directly indicate a change in any specific component. Weight cannot be used in isolation to assess nutritional status in children with neurodisability.

Table 6.1 shows the different weighing equipment and methods commonly used. There are no studies comparing the different methods of weight measurement. In a group of

53 children with neurodisability, we found that repeat weight measurements taken on two separate occasions 2–4 weeks apart showed a TEM for weight of 0.55kg for standers and 0.75kg for non-standers (Hardy et al. 2018).

Height

For many children with neurological impairment, height/length measurement is very challenging. For children who can stand, height can be measured using a stadiometer.

For children who are unable to stand with CP, supine length has been measured using a rollameter or digital supine measuring table (Samson-Fang & Stevenson 2000). However, we found using a rollameter in a group of non-standers with neurological impairment did not achieve good reliability (TEM 2.47cm) (Hardy et al. 2018).

Haapala et al. (2015) tested the reliability of a supine length from summed segmental measurements in a small group of children who were able to stand and lie recumbent. The four continuous segments were (1) from the top of the head to the acromion process; (2) acromion process of the shoulder to the greater trochanter of the hip; (3) greater trochanter of the hip to the lateral joint of the knee; (4) knee joint line to the bottom of the heel. The agreement between standing height and recumbent length was satisfactory (Haapala et al. 2015).

In order to overcome the difficulties associated with supine length measurement, a number of different equations have been developed to predict height from a segmental measure (Chumlea et al. 1994; Stevenson 1995; Gauld et al. 2004). Segmental measurements including knee height, tibial length, upper arm length and ulnar length have been used to estimate supine length.

Knee height has been measured in children aged 0–12 years with CP with good intra- and interobserver reliability reported by Stevenson (1995). In his original cohort used to develop the equations, children with severe contractures and scoliosis were excluded from the sample. Estimated height from knee height showed better agreement with measured supine length than tibia length or upper arm length (Stevenson 1995) (Fig. 6.1). The Gauld et al. (2004) knee height equation was developed from a cohort of neurotypical children.

The difference between the measured supine length and that estimated from these equations has been tested using Bland–Altman limits of agreement (Haapala et al. 2015). Height estimation from the Chumlea et al. (1994) knee height equation deteriorated as the height increased. Stevenson's (1995) knee height equation underestimated the measured supine length but performed better for children with milder disability (GMFCS I–III) than for children with GMFCS IV–V. They showed that this equation predicted the supine length better than the Gauld et al. (2004) ulna equation which tended to

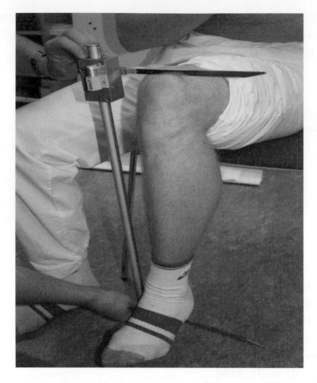

Figure 6.1 Measurement of knee height using calipers. (Courtesy of Magnus Dahlseng and Ane Finbråten.)

Table 6.2 Equations to predict supine length from knee height (Adapted from Haapala et al. 2015)

Stevenson (1995) Age 0–12 years	
Knee height	H = (2.68 × KH) + 24.2
Tibia length	H = (3.26 × TL) + 30.8
Gauld et al. (2004) Age 7+ years	
Males	
Knee height	H = 2.423KH + 1.327A + 21.818
Tibia length	H = 2.758T + 1.717A + 36.509
Females	
Knee height	H = 2.473KH + 1.187A + 21.151
Tibia length	H = 2.771T + 1.457A + 37.748
H = estimated height, KH = knee height, A = age, T = tibia length	

overestimate by a wide margin. Stevenson's (1995) tibial length predictive equation consistently underestimated supine length, with differences as wide as –2.91cm (+/– 5.91cm).

Haapala et al. (2015) concludes that although segmental measures are repeatable, their use in equations predicts height with only poor to moderate agreement. Therefore, when an estimation of height is required, for children less than 12 years, the Stevenson (1995) equation can be used, and for individuals over 7 years, the equation published by Gauld et al. (2004) may be appropriate, particularly for individuals with GMFCS IV–V (see Table 6.2).

As a measure of supine length, a summed segmental measurement overcomes the limitations of contractures and disproportionate lower extremity growth (Haapala et al. 2015).

Body Mass Index

BMI – calculated as weight/height^2 – is widely used to describe the index of relative weight. Although its correlation with clinical outcomes is established in adults, the predictive value (morbidity and mortality) is less clear in children, particularly those with neurological impairment.

BMI can be confounded by inaccurate measurement – particularly of height/length, and this is a further risk factor for poor validity in these children. In our observations, BMI showed poor TEM for non-standers (1.37kg/m^2), as a result of the difficulties in measuring height (Hardy et al. 2018). The TEM for BMI of standers was 0.33kg/m^2, with a lower TEM for height measurement in this group (Hardy et al. 2018).

BMI does not describe body composition. Although it may be intuitive to correct a weight according to height, using the BMI to assess body composition can be misleading in children with neurological impairment, especially CP (Samson-Fang & Stevenson 2000; Kuperminc et al. 2010). Although BMI has been shown to perform well in predicting body fat in children who have excess fat, it underestimates body fat in children who have a low BMI; for example 'malnourished' in terms of BMI may actually have an increase in relative body fat and a severe decrease in lean tissue (Wells & Fewtrell 2006; Kuperminc et al. 2010).

Kuperminc et al. (2010) compared percentage body fat using dual X-ray absorptiometry (DXA) with BMI in a group of children with CP. In children who had been identified as carrying excess weight from DXA, only 19% were recognised as having excess fat with the BMI alone.

Children with neurological impairment attending specialist support schools show a greater prevalence of overweight and obesity compared with mainstream schools (Stewart et al. 2009; Abeysekara et al. 2014). There are a number of reasons for this, including overnutrition and limited mobility; however, some syndromic conditions may also contribute to excess weight gain.

Interpretation of Measurements

Patterns of human growth are predictable in the typically developing population (Day et al. 2007). Growth reference charts have been constructed for healthy children and are used as a standard clinical tool in many countries with local variations (UK-WHO growth charts, USA-CDC growth chart). For neurologically impaired children, no one set of disease-specific reference standards exist.

Growth in Cerebral Palsy

The majority of research on longitudinal growth has been conducted on children with CP. Stallings et al. (1993) recognised that growth in children with CP was affected by severity of the condition and nutrition, as well as genetics, sex, race and pubertal status. It was found that nutritional status explained 10–15% of the variation in growth, but the main influences on growth were the variables associated with severity of the condition.

Strand et al. (2016) studied children with CP from birth and found reduced growth in the first 5 years of life in children who were more severely affected and who had feeding difficulties. Children who were born small for gestational age (SGA) also had reduced growth including head circumference growth which decreased during the first year of life. Normal longitudinal growth was seen in non-SGA children and children without feeding difficulties, even if they were severely impaired.

Linear growth in children with CP is also affected by the underlying neurological deficit which affects the neuromuscular bone unit. Haapala et al. (2015) found the ratio of ulna length to knee height was greater in patients with GMFCS IV–V than in GMFCS I–III, implying hypoplastic growth in the distal lower limb.

Day et al. (2007) constructed height, weight and BMI charts stratified by motor and feeding skills – again showing that the most severely affected have the poorest growth and greater morbidity (see Appendix A). Children with the best mobility had weight centiles equivalent with the general population. There is progressive deviation from the general population reference as functional ability deteriorates; the most severely affected group (not gastrostomy-fed) had weights below the 10th centile for the general population, with medians more than 20% below from as early as 2 years. It is important to note that the most severe group who were fed by tube had better weight centiles than those who were not.

At puberty, weight in the moderate to severely affected group increases more slowly than the usual rapid weight gain seen in neurotypical children (Day et al. 2007).

Day et al. (2007) showed height followed a similar pattern to weight. For the least severely affected group the curves were similar to the general population with a characteristic earlier growth for females (pubertal growth spurt) but with heights of males overtaking females at age 20.

The North American Growth in Cerebral Palsy Project acknowledged the difficulties associated with measuring supine length in those who are more severely affected and measured knee height and upper arm length with a standardised technique as proxies for growth (Stevenson et al. 2006). They constructed growth charts for knee height, upper arm length, skinfolds and weight.

In this group of more severely affected children, the children were smaller, thinner and lighter than their typically developing peers and this is more pronounced as they age. Where the knee height curves overlap with the centiles of typically developing children, at adolescence none of those with CP were above the 5th centile. The usual adolescent growth spurt was blunted.

Are CP Growth Charts for Height, Weight and BMI Clinically Useful?

The main concern is that the charts produced by The Life Expectancy Project (Day et al. 2007) from the cohort of children in California are a descriptive reference of how a particular group of children grew rather than a prescriptive standard of how they 'should' grow. Defining a 'healthy' population of children with CP may not be possible or appropriate (Brooks et al. 2011).

The North American Growth in Cerebral Palsy Project acknowledged that their charts were not produced as a reference to show ideal growth trajectories (Stevenson et al. 2006). Instead they correlated better knee length growth with less use of healthcare services and greater participation in usual activities. It is not known whether children who grow better are healthier, or if children who are healthier grow better.

Brooks et al. (2011) argue that growth charts should aim to identify children with CP who are at greater risk of morbidity and mortality. A total of 25 545 children aged 2–20 years with CP were analysed to determine (low) weight thresholds that are associated with increased risk of morbidity and mortality. Weight-for-age centiles were constructed, with a shaded area indicating the threshold at which there is greater risk of nutritional and health morbidity (www.lifeexpectancy.org).

Comorbidity was more common among those with weights below the 20th centile in GMFCS I–V (without tube feeds). For GMFCS I–II weights below the 5th centile were associated with a mortality hazard ratio of 2.2 and for III–V weights below 20th centile were associated with a hazard ratio of 1.5.

One of the main limitations of The Life Expectancy Project is that the cohort weights were not always measured directly but some were reported from parents (Day et al. 2007; Brooks et al. 2011). Discrepancies between weights recorded by the evaluator and those in the child's medical record were found in 9% of a random sample.

There is no description of a standardised technique for height or length measurement in this cohort (Day et al. 2007). However, the authors acknowledge the difficulty of measuring height in children with significant motor impairment and suggest that the height curves for groups GMFCS IV–V should be viewed with caution.

ARE THE AMERICAN CP GROWTH CHARTS APPLICABLE INTERNATIONALLY?

Araújo and Silva (2013) evaluated anthropometric data of a cohort of 187 Brazilian children with CP aged 2–16 in relation to general population reference (CDC) curves and the curves described by Brooks et al. (2007). In this cohort, 56% had weights below the 50th centile for the Brooks et al. (2007) curves and 86% below the 50th centile for the CDC reference.

Using the definition of nutritionally at risk of a weight <10th centile on the Brooks et al. (2007) charts 10% of the Brazilian sample were at risk. If the CDC < 10th centile was used, then 51% of individuals were defined as at risk. Araújo and Silva (2013) suggest that using charts for typically developing children in a population with neurodisability overestimates those at risk of undernutrition.

Wright et al. (2017) compared weights, heights and BMI for 195 Scottish children with CP between 1997 and 2013 with the data from The Life Expectancy Project cohort in California and the UK-WHO charts (Freeman et al. 1995; Day et al. 2007; Brooks et al. 2011).

Using the UK-WHO reference, height and weight z-scores decreased with age with median height z-scores close to the 2nd centile. There was poor 'fit' for height for GMFCS II–V and for weight at levels IV–V and this was present from 2 years. However, for the CP reference (Brooks et al. 2011), the 'fit' was good for all GMFCS levels for weight, height and BMI except for levels III and V. Overall, the children in the UK tended to be taller compared to the American CP charts at all GMFCS levels (Wright et al. 2017).

APPLICATION OF GROWTH CHARTS IN NEUROLOGICALLY IMPAIRED CHILDREN

The use of CP-specific growth charts remains controversial. The fundamental argument is whether it is possible to define a reference population – that is, what is 'normal', 'healthy' growth for a child with CP. European Society for Paediatric Gastroenterology Hepatology and Nutrition (ESPGHAN) guidelines do not recommend the use of CP-specific growth charts to identify undernutrition (Romano et al. 2017). Future research may focus on understanding the reasons for the deviation of growth from neurotypical children with age and severity, as described in the current CP-specific growth charts.

Amongst children with neurological impairment, there are many who have syndromic conditions that affect growth. Other charts describing the growth of neurologically impaired children (such as Down syndrome or Sotos syndrome) are available and the Down syndrome medical interest group recommends their use (Styles et al. 2002).

APPLICATION OF PREDICTIVE EQUATIONS FROM ANTHROPOMETRIC MEASURES IN NEUROLOGICALLY IMPAIRED CHILDREN

Measurements of supine length are challenging in all neurologically impaired children, and repeatability is poor – particularly in children unable to stand. This will clearly affect the interpretation of a single measurement in time and therefore serial measurements are needed, using standardised techniques.

ESPGHAN guidelines recommend measuring knee height or tibial length to assess linear growth when height cannot be measured. Although measurement of knee height has shown good repeatability, this is not translated in its ability to predict supine length, except in children under 12 years of age (see Table 6.2). It is suggested that serial measurements of knee height or tibial length should be taken to monitor growth, although reference data for 'ideal' growth in knee height are not available. The only descriptive data comes from the North American Growth in Cerebral Palsy Project (Stevenson et al. 2006).

Skinfolds and Circumferences

ESPGHAN recommends that the assessment of nutritional status in children with neurological impairment should not be based solely on weight and height measurements (Romano et al. 2017). Assessment of body composition gives a better guide to nutritional status than body weight alone (Wells & Fewtrell 2006). Various simple anthropometric measurements are available in the clinical setting, including skinfolds, mid-upper arm circumference (MUAC) and waist circumference. Some of these measures can be interpreted either by using reference charts or used in equations to predict body fat percentage. Evaluation of the predictive equations has been conducted against various body component reference models; however, many of the assumptions made in the predictive equations have their own intrinsic flaws (Wells & Fewtrell 2006).

SKINFOLDS

Common sites chosen for skinfold measurements are arms – triceps and biceps, and trunk – subscapular and supra-iliac (Fig. 6.2). Different techniques for locating landmarks and the position of the calipers have been described (Tanner & Whitehouse 1975; Stewart et al. 2011). Until an international consensus is obtained, it is important that standardised protocols are established locally and quality assurance measures are in place.

Tanner and Whitehouse (1975) developed triceps and subscapular skinfold reference charts by age and sex on a sample of typically developing British children. These references have been converted to standard deviation scores (z-scores) to allow a convenient comparison over time (Davies et al. 1993). In the USA, triceps skinfold reference tables were developed from the National Health and Nutrition Examination Survey 1 (Frisancho 1981) (see Appendix B).

Predictive Techniques

Skinfolds have also been used to predict body fat percentage from two or more measurements. Validation of a number of different equations have shown both over- and underestimation of body fat percentage in typically developing children when compared to body fat percentage calculated from underwater weighing as the reference method (Reilly et al. 1995). Slaughter et al. (1988) developed a predictive equation

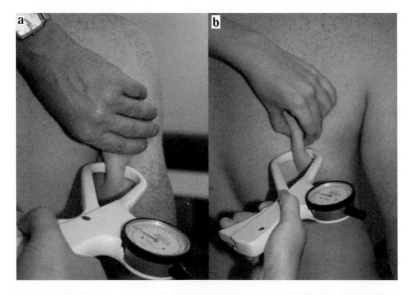

Figure 6.2 a: Measurement of triceps skinfold thickness using calipers. b: Measurement of subscapular skinfold thickness using calipers. (Courtesy of Magnus Dahlseng and Ane Finbråten.)

which accounted for race, age, sex and pubertal status. These equations have performed well in predicting percentage body fat against DXA as the reference method in neurotypical children (Steinberger et al. 2005), but have consistently underestimated percentage body fat in children with CP as compared with DXA or deuterium dilution technique (Stallings et al. 1995; van den Berg-Emons et al. 1998; Liu et al. 2005; Gurka et al. 2010). It remains unclear why Slaughter's equation underestimates percentage body fat in children with CP. It has been suggested that children with CP have relatively large internal (intra-abdominal) rather than peripheral fat stores (van den Berg-Emons et al. 1998; Kuperminc et al. 2010).

Gurka et al. (2010) developed corrections to the original Slaughter equations validated against DXA using a population of children aged 8–18 with CP, which accounted for GMFCS level in addition. Finbråten et al. (2015) confirmed the reliability of Gurka's CP-specific equation. See Appendix C for the equations. However, using BIA and D_2O dilution as the reference method, Rieken et al. (2011) found that the CP-specific equation tended to overestimate percentage body fat.

It has been argued that the use of predictive equations is inherently flawed as they confound the accurate raw values with an error from the prediction itself (standard error of the estimate) (Wells & Fewtrell 2006). It has therefore been suggested that raw skinfolds (or their SDS) are reliable indices of regional fatness, and when measured serially could provide an indication of fatness.

CIRCUMFERENCES

Mid-upper Arm Circumference

MUAC has been used to assist identification of nutritional status, either alone or in combination with triceps skinfolds (Craig et al. 2014; Mramba et al. 2017).

MUAC and triceps skinfolds have been used together to predict upper arm fat mass and upper arm lean mass (Frisancho 1981). This measurement is based on the assumption that the upper arm is cylindrical, the subcutaneous fat is evenly distributed round a central core of muscle, the triceps accurately separates fat and lean components and represents twice the thickness of subcutaneous fat in the arm. The muscle area does not take into account the humeral diameter. Predicting the cross-sectional area of fat gives little more information than triceps skinfolds alone (Chomtho et al. 2006).

Furthermore, using MUAC and triceps skinfold to predict upper arm lean mass shows only moderate correlation when compared with DXA.

Children with CP have been found to have lower overall MUAC, triceps skinfold and mid-upper arm fat area compared with typically developing children (Kuperminc et al.

2010). Peripheral measurements (MUAC or triceps skinfolds) are unlikely to accurately predict overall fat levels in children with CP, particularly because these children can have increased intra-abdominal fat stores (Kuperminc et al. 2010).

Waist Circumferences

In neurotypical children, waist circumference has been used successfully as a simple measure of central fatness (Wells & Fewtrell 2006). However, in our observations this is difficult to achieve reliably in children with neurodisability: true waist circumference showed a TEM of 1.82cm and 1.86cm in non-standers and standers respectively; umbilical waist circumference showed a TEM of 1.83cm and 2.04cm in non-standers and standers respectively (Hardy et al. 2018).

Body Composition

Using a two-compartment model of body composition, fat mass is often expressed as a percentage of total weight. However, this does not reflect the contribution of fat-free (lean) mass; for example, a child with a low fat-free mass may have a high fat mass percentage, despite a normal or low fat mass (Wells 2001). In order to express body composition to account for this, it is suggested that both fat-free mass and fat mass should be expressed as an index relative to height^2 (Wells 2001).

Bioelectrical Impedance Analysis

Bioelectrical impedance analysis (BIA) measures the resistance or impedance of the body to a small electrical current. Lean tissue contains a high level of water and electrolytes and therefore acts as an electrical conductor. In practice, using BIA requires applying equations to predict total body water, which is then converted to fat-free mass. BIA offers the clinician a simple, non-invasive method of measuring fat-free mass. Fat mass can then be predicted by subtracting fat-free mass from weight.

Fat-free mass and fat mass estimates from BIA use equations that are population specific and perform poorly in healthy individuals when evaluated against reference methods (Wells et al. 1999; Parker et al. 2003) with errors typically +/– 8% fat. This may reflect the limitation of the regression equations used which were developed on small numbers of children over a wide age range. Total values of lean and fat mass are hard to interpret in isolation as both vary in relation to height (Wright et al. 2008). Wright et al. (2008) used BIA data from a large UK cohort of typically developing children and then applied these to a small population of children with neurodisability, including some who were gastrostomy fed. Overall, the children with neurodisability were short and had low to average BMIs compared to their neurotypical peers. BIA showed these children had low lean mass indices and yet had fat indices that were close to the reference population (Wright et al. 2008).

Feasibility studies conducted on children with CP have shown BIA to be achievable and reliable (Veugelers et al. 2006; Wright et al. 2008). Bell et al. (2013) evaluated three different equations for estimation of total body water in children under the age of 4 with CP using deuterium dilution technique as the reference. Estimates of total body water were most accurate using the Fjeld equation for both children with bilateral impairment and unilateral impairment when measured on the unimpaired side (Bell et al. 2013).

BIA may be easier to achieve than skinfolds in 'standers' (Hardy et al. 2018). The reliability of BIA is affected by differing states of hydration and so may be less reliable in children with greater degree of neurological impairment.

If used with understanding of the limitations of the method, BIA could make an important contribution to body composition measurement as a measure of total body water and fat-free (lean) mass. Further research should focus on the most appropriate body composition models and predictive equations in these children.

Dual-energy X-ray Absorptiometry

DXA was originally used to assess bone mineral mass in adults with osteoporosis. It relies on the differential absorption of X-rays of two different energies. The process quantifies the overlying soft tissue and values of fat and fat-free mass are also calculated.

Whole-body DXA has become the 'criterion standard' for the measurement of body composition in research studies, and can be used for children and infants.

One of the difficulties in using DXA is that although the technique can easily analyse proportions of fat and tissues in the limbs, it is more difficult in the trunk because the pelvis, spine and ribs substantially obscure the pixels, making soft tissue estimation less accurate. In lean individuals, fewer soft tissue pixels are available for estimation of adjacent pixels which reduces accuracy (Wells & Fewtrell 2006).

DXA is widely used to assess bone mineral density at the lumbar spine, hip and femur in children with neurological impairment. Low bone mineralisation is seen in neurologically impaired children with limited mobility, feeding difficulties, antiepileptic drugs, lower fat mass and previous fractures (Bianchi et al. 2014). Bone mineral density z-scores <–2 as measured by DXA showed a prevalence of more than 70% in children with severe neurological impairment, with an annual incidence of fractures of 4% (Bianchi et al. 2014). In order to identify those at increased risk of fracture, the International Society for Clinical Densitometry recommends assessing bone mineral density at the lateral distal femur site in children with neurological impairment as this is the most common site of fractures in non-ambulant children (Bianchi et al. 2014).

RED FLAGS

There are no strict criteria to define undernutrition in children with neurodisability, owing to the complexities of measuring and interpreting anthropometric data as described above.

ESPGHAN guidelines suggest the use of one or more of the following red flag warning signs to identify undernutrition in children with neurological impairment (Romano et al. 2017):

1. Weight-for-age z-score <–2

2. Triceps skinfold thickness <10th centile for age and sex

3. Mid-upper arm fat or muscle area <10th centile

4. Faltering weight and/or failure to thrive

5. Physical signs of undernutrition such as decubitis ulcers and poor peripheral circulation

The National Institute for Health and Care Excellence (2017) definition of failure to thrive (faltering growth) using the UK-WHO growth charts is:

• A fall across one or more weight centile spaces, if birthweight was below the 9th centile

• A fall across two or more weight centile spaces, if birthweight was between the 9th and 91st centiles

• A fall across three or more weight centile spaces, if birthweight was above the 91st centile

• When current weight is below the 2nd centile for age, whatever the birthweight

For reference:

Weight-for-age charts (UK): https://www.rcpch.ac.uk/growthcharts

Weight-for-age charts (CDC): https://www.cdc.gov/growthcharts/clinical_charts.htm

CONCLUSION

Anthropometric measures provide us with tools to assess the extent to which physiological and metabolic demands for energy and nutrients are being satisfied. They give us an indication of whether the child is in energy balance (positive or negative), whether intervention is required and help to monitor the success of the intervention.

This chapter has explored various measurement techniques available in practice, and highlights the difficulties in the measurement itself and the interpretation of the measures in the neurologically impaired child. Understanding the sources of variation in any choice of measurement for use in clinical or community settings may help reduce errors and improve reliability of these measurements. The limitations we have presented should in no way undermine the importance of regularly monitoring this group of vulnerable children.

Future research may focus on how anthropometric measurements relate not only to growth and development but also to the metabolic health of children with neurological impairment.

REFERENCES

Abeysekara P, Turchi R, O'Neil M (2014) Obesity and children with special healthcare needs: special considerations for a special population. *Curr Opin Pediatr* 26(4): 508–515. doi: 10.1097/ MOP.0000000000000124.

Araújo LA, Silva LR (2013) Anthropometric assessment of patients with cerebral palsy: which curves are more appropriate? *J Pediatr* 89(3): 307–314. doi: 10.1016/j.jped.2012.11.008.

Bell KL, Boyd RN, Walker JL, Stevenson RD, Davies PS (2013) The use of bioelectrical impedance analysis to estimate total body water in young children with cerebral palsy. *Clin Nutr* 32(4): 579–584. doi: 10.1016/j.clnu.2012.10.005.

Bianchi ML, Leonard MB, Bechtold S et al. (2014) Bone health in children and adolescents with chronic diseases that may affect the skeleton: the 2013 ISCD Pediatric Official Positions. *J Clin Densitom* 17(2): 281–294. doi: 10.1016/j.jocd.2014.01.005.

Brooks J, Day S, Shavelle R, Strauss D (2011) Low weight, morbidity, and mortality in children with cerebral palsy: new clinical growth charts. *Pediatrics* 128(2): e299–307. doi: 10.1542/ peds.2010-2801.

Chomtho S, Fewtrell MS, Jaffe A, Williams JE, Wells JC (2006) Evaluation of arm anthropometry for assessing pediatric body composition: evidence from healthy and sick children. *Pediatr Res* 59(6): 860–865. doi: 10.1203/01.pdr.0000219395.83159.91.

Chumlea WC, Guo SS, Steinbaugh ML (1994) Prediction of stature from knee height for black and white adults and children with application to mobility-impaired or handicapped persons. *J Am Diet Assoc* 94(12): 1385–1388. doi: https://doi.org/10.1016/0002-8223(94)92540-2.

Craig E, Bland R, Ndirangu J, Reilly JJ (2014) Use of mid-upper arm circumference for determining overweight and overfatness in children and adolescents. *Arch Dis Child* 99: 763–766. doi: 10.1136/archdischild-2013-305137.

Davies PS, Day JM, Cole TJ (1993) Converting Tanner-Whitehouse reference tricep and subscapular skinfold measurements to standard deviation scores. *Eur J Clin Nutr* 47(8): 559–566.

Day SM, Strauss DJ, Vachon PJ, Rosenbloom L, Shavelle RM, Wu YW (2007) Growth patterns in a population of children and adolescents with cerebral palsy. *Dev Med Child Neurol* 49(3): 167–171. doi: 10.1111/j.1469-8749.2007.00167.x.

de Onis M, Onyango AW, Van den Broeck J, Chumlea WC, Martorell R (2004) Measurement and standardization protocols for anthropometry used in the construction of a new international growth reference. *Food Nutr Bull* 25(Suppl 1): S27–36. doi: 10.1177/15648265040251S104.

Finbråten AK, Martins C, Andersen GL et al. (2015) Assessment of body composition in children with cerebral palsy: a cross-sectional study in Norway. *Dev Med Child Neurol* 57(9): 858–864. doi: 10.1111/dmcn.12752.

Freeman JV, Cole TJ, Chinn S, Jones PR, White EM, Preece MA (1995) Cross sectional stature and weight reference curves for the UK, 1990. *Arch Dis Child* 73(1): 17–24. doi: http://dx.doi.org/10.1136/adc.73.1.17.

Frisancho AR (1981) New norms of upper limb fat and muscle areas for assessment of nutritional status. *Am J Clin Nutr* 34(11): 2540–2545.

Gauld LM, Kappers J, Carlin JB, Robertson CF (2004) Height prediction from ulna length. *Dev Med Child Neurol* 46(7): 475-480. doi: 10.1111/j.1469-8749.2004.tb00508.x.

Gurka MJ, Kuperminc MN, Busby MG et al. (2010) Assessment and correction of skinfold thickness equations in estimating body fat in children with cerebral palsy. *Dev Med Child Neurol* 52(2): e35-41. doi: 10.1111/j.1469-8749.2009.03474.x.

Haapala H, Peterson MD, Daunter A, Hurvitz EA (2015) Agreement between actual height and estimated height using segmental limb lengths for individuals with cerebral palsy. *Am J Phys Med Rehabil* 94(7): 539–546. doi: 10.1097/PHM.0000000000000205.

Hardy J, Kuter H, Campbell M. et al. (2018) Reliability of anthropometric measurements in children with special needs. *Arch Dis Child* 103: 757–762.

Kuperminc MN, Gurka MJ, Bennis JA et al. (2010) Anthropometric measures: poor predictors of body fat in children with moderate to severe cerebral palsy. *Dev Med Child Neurol* 52(9): 824–830. doi: 10.1111/j.1469-8749.2010.03694.x.

Liu LF, Roberts R, Moyer-Mileur L, Samson-Fang L (2005) Determination of body composition in children with cerebral palsy: bioelectrical impedance analysis and anthropometry vs dual-energy x-ray absorptiometry. *J Am Diet Assoc* 105(5): 794–797. doi: https://doi.org/10.1016/j.jada.2005.02.006.

Morris C, Janssens A, Tomlinson R, Williams J, Logan S (2013) Towards a definition of neurodisability: a Delphi survey. *Dev Med Child Neurol* 55(12): 1103–1108. doi: 10.1111/dmcn.12218.

Mramba L, Ngari M, Mwangome M et al. (2017) A growth reference for mid upper arm circumference for age among school age children and adolescents, and validation for mortality: growth curve construction and longitudinal cohort study. *BMJ* 358: j3423. doi: 10.1136/bmj.j3423.

Parker L, Reilly JJ, Slater C, Wells JC, Pitsiladis Y (2003) Validity of six field and laboratory methods for measurement of body composition in boys. *Obes Res* 11(7): 852–858. doi: 10.1038/oby.2003.117.

Reilly T, Tyrrell A, Troup JD (1984) Circadian variation in human stature. *Chronobiol Int* 1(2): 121–126.

Reilly JJ, Wilson J, Durnin JV (1995) Determination of body composition from skinfold thickness: a validation study. *Arch Dis Child* 73(4): 305–310.

Rieken R, van Goudoever JB, Schierbeek H et al. (2011) Measuring body composition and energy expenditure in children with severe neurologic impairment and intellectual disability. *Am J Clin Nutr* 94(3): 759–766. doi: 10.3945/ajcn.110.003798.

Romano C, van Wynckel M, Hulst J et al. (2017) European Society for Paediatric Gastroenterology, Hepatology and Nutrition guidelines for the evaluation and treatment of gastrointestinal and nutritional complications in children with neurological impairment. *J Pediatr Gastroent Nutr* 65(2): 242–264. doi: 10.1097/MPG.0000000000001646.

Samson-Fang LJ, Stevenson RD (2000) Identification of malnutrition in children with cerebral palsy: poor performance of weight-for-height centiles. *Dev Med Child Neurol* 42(3): 162–168. doi: 10.1111/j.1469-8749.2000.tb00064.x.

Slaughter MH, Lohman TG, Boileau RA et al. (1988) Skinfold equations for estimation of body fatness in children and youth. *Hum Biol* 60(5): 709–723.

Stallings VA, Charney EB, Davies JC, Cronk CE (1993) Nutritional status and growth of children with diplegic or hemiplegic cerebral palsy. *Dev Med Child Neurol* 35(11): 997–1006. doi: 10.1111/j.1469-8749.1993.tb11582.x.

Stallings VA, Cronk CE, Zemel BS, Charney EB (1995) Body composition in children with spastic quadriplegic cerebral palsy. *J Pediatr* 126(5Pt1): 833–839. doi: https://doi.org/10.1016/S0022-3476(95)70424-8.

Steinberger J, Jacobs DR, Raatz S, Moran A, Hong CP, Sinaiko AR (2005) Comparison of body fatness measurements by BMI and skinfolds vs dual energy X-ray absorptiometry and their relation to cardiovascular risk factors in adolescents. *Int J Obes* 29(11): 1346–1352. doi: 10.1038/sj.ijo.0803026.

Stevenson RD (1995) Use of segmental measures to estimate stature in children with cerebral palsy. *Arch Pediatr Adolesc Med* 149(6): 658–662. doi:10.1001/archpedi.1995.02170190068012.

Stevenson RD, Conaway M, Chumlea WC et al. (2006) Growth and health in children with moderate-to-severe cerebral palsy. *Pediatrics* 118(3): 1010–1018. doi: 10.1542/peds.2006-0298.

Stewart LM et al. (2009) High risk group: children with special needs. Audit reported at the 4th annual paediatric study day, Manchester 2009.

Stewart A, Marfell-Jones M, Olds T, de Ridder H (2011) *International Standards for Anthropometric Assessment*. Lower Hutt, New Zealand: ISAK.

Strand KM, Dahlseng MO, Lydersen S et al. (2016) Growth during infancy and early childhood in children with cerebral palsy: a population-based study. *Dev Med Child Neurol* 58(9): 924–930. doi: 10.1111/dmcn.13098.

Styles ME, Cole TJ, Dennis J, Preece MA (2002) New cross sectional stature, weight, and head circumference references for Down's syndrome in the UK and Republic of Ireland. *Arch Dis Child* 87(2): 104–108.

Tanner JM, Whitehouse RH (1975) Revised standards for triceps and subscapular skinfolds in British children. *Arch Dis Child* 50(2): 142–145.

van den Berg-Emons RJ, van Baak MA, Westerterp KR (1998) Are skinfold measurements suitable to compare body fat between children with spastic cerebral palsy and healthy controls? *Dev Med Child Neurol* 40(5): 335–339. doi: 10.1111/j.1469-8749.1998.tb15385.x.

Veugelers R, Penning C, van Gulik ME, Tibboel D, Evenhuis HM (2006) Feasibility of bioelectrical impedance analysis in children with a severe generalized cerebral palsy. *Nutrition* 22(1): 16–22. doi: https://doi.org/10.1016/j.nut.2005.05.005.

Wells JC, Fuller NJ, Dewit O, Fewtrell MS, Elia M, Cole TJ (1999) Four component model of body composition in children: density and hydration of fat free mass and comparison with simpler models. *Am J Clin Nutr* 69(5): 904–912.

Wells JC (2001) A critique of the expression of paediatric body composition data. *Arch Dis Child* 85(1): 67–72. doi: 10.1136/adc.85.1.67.

Wells JC, Fewtrell MS (2006) Measuring body composition. *Arch Dis Child* 91(7): 612–617. doi: 10.1136/adc.2005.085522.

Wootton S, Durkin K, Jackson A (2014) Quality control issues related to assessment of body composition. *Food Nutr Bull* 35(Suppl 2): S79–85. doi: 10.1177/15648265140352S112.

Wright CM, Sherriff A, Ward SC, McColl JH, Reilly JJ, Ness AR (2008) Development of bioelectrical impedance-derived indices of fat and fat-free mass for assessment of nutritional status in childhood. *Eur J Clin Nutr* 62(2): 210–217. doi:10.1038/sj.ejcn.1602714.

Wright CM, Reynolds L, Ingram E, Cole TJ, Brooks J (2017) Validation of US cerebral palsy growth charts using a UK cohort. *Dev Med Child Neurol* 59(9): 933–938. doi: 10.1111/dmcn.13495.

APPENDIX A

Descriptive growth charts for children with cerebral palsy can be found at the following link: http://lifeexpectancy.org/articles/NewGrowthCharts.shtml.

APPENDIX B

The following reference describes how to calculate SDS (z-scores) for tricep and subscapular skinfolds using the LMS method (tables and equations included) based on the original Tanner and Whitehouse British cohort (1975):

Davies PS, Day JM, Cole TJ (1993) Converting Tanner–Whitehouse reference tricep and subscapular skinfold measurements to standard deviation scores. *Eur J Clin Nutr* 47: 559–566.

For the under 5s the WHO standards for triceps and subscapular centiles and SDS can be found at the following link:

http://www.who.int/childgrowth/standards/second_set/technical_report_2.pdf.

This reference also includes head circumference and arm circumference.

The following reference gives tables of skinfold thickness, midupper arm fat and muscle areas and the equations used to predict this from data collected in the USA:

Frisancho AR (1981) New norms of upper limb fat and muscle areas for assessment of nutritional status. *Am J Clin Nutr* 34(11): 2540–2545.

APPENDIX C

See Table 6.3 for predictive equations for percentage body fat in children using triceps and subscapular skinfold with correction for cerebral palsy (Gurkha et al. 2010).

Table 6.3 Original Slaughter equations and corrections for children with cerebral palsy. (Reprinted from Gurka et al. 2010 with permission from Mac Keith Press.)

Population	Original Slaughter equations for predicting percentage body fat[7]
Sum (triceps, subscapular) ≤35mm	
Males	
Prepubescent[a] white	% Body fat = 1.21(tri + sub) − 0.008(tri + sub)^2 − 1.7
Prepubescent black	% Body fat = 1.21(tri + sub) − 0.008(tri + sub)^2 − 3.2
Pubescent white	% Body fat = 1.21(tri + sub) − 0.008(tri + sub)^2 − 3.4
Pubescent black	% Body fat = 1.21(tri + sub) − 0.008(tri + sub)^2 − 5.2
Postpubescent white	% Body fat = 1.21(tri + sub) − 0.008(tri + sub)^2 − 5.5
Postpubescent black	% Body fat = 1.21(tri + sub) − 0.008(tri + sub)^2 − 6.8
Females (all)	% Body fat = 1.33(tri + sub) − 0.013(tri + sub)^2 − 2.5
Sum (triceps, subscapular) >35mm	
Males (all)	% Body fat = 0.783(tri + sub) + 1.6
Females (all)	% Body fat = 0.546(tri + sub) + 9.7
	Cerebral-palsy-specific corrections to Slaughter-estimated percentage body fat[b]
Overall correction	+12.2
Additional correction for	
Males	−5.0
More severe GMFCS	+5.1
Black race	−3.1
Pubescent	+2.0
Postpubescent	−4.6
Sum (triceps, subscapular) > 35mm	−3.2

[a]Prepubescent, Tanner stage 1,2; pubescent, Tanner stage 3; postpubescent, Tanner stage 4, 5.
[b]Instructions for using these corrections on a given child with CP: always add 12.2 to the Slaughter-estimated percentage body fat. Then, if the individual falls within each of the additional categories, add that respective corrections as well. For example, for a black pubescent male at GMFCS level 1 whose sum (triceps, subscapular) <35mm, the predicted percentage body fat = Slaughter percentage body fat +12.2−5.0−3.1+2.0. Tri + sub, triceps skinfold + subscapular skinfold GMFCS, Gross Motor Function Classification System.

CHAPTER 7

Assessment of Nutritional State: Dietetic, Energy and Macronutrients

Jacqueline L Walker and Kristie L Bell

INTRODUCTION

Nutritional assessment is an essential component of comprehensive management and care for children with neurological impairment (NI), as nutrition concerns can be common (Kuperminc & Stevenson 2008). As noted in previous chapters, maintaining adequate growth can be a challenge. Poor growth and malnutrition have been linked to poorer health, decreased motor function, decreased survival, increased healthcare utilisation and lower participation in usual daily activities (Stevenson et al. 2006; Brooks et al. 2011). Nutritional factors that help explain the aetiology of suboptimal growth include inadequate dietary intake (energy, macronutrient and micronutrient intake), altered energy requirements and poor nutritional status (Hogan 2004; Kuperminc & Stevenson 2008). Nutrition concerns are more common in children with feeding and swallowing difficulties; motor, physical or sensory impairments; and behavioural difficulties (Sullivan et al. 2002; Stevenson et al. 2006; Vernon-Roberts et al. 2010; Oftedal et al. 2017). Because of these complexities, nutritional assessment of children with NI is not straightforward. It is essential that the array of factors involved is considered as part of regular clinical practices. This will then inform the nutritional management strategies used, and ensure that care is individualised (Sullivan et al. 2002). By maximising nutritional status, clinicians can ensure that children are growing adequately, which in turn will help maintain a good quality of life for both children and families.

The assessment of dietary intake in combination with an understanding of nutritional requirements will assist in identifying if children are meeting their daily energy and nutrient requirements. Positive energy balance is required for weight gain and optimal growth and development. Extended periods of neutral energy balance for a child will result in inadequate weight gain and growth. Negative energy balance will result in weight loss. Both neutral and negative energy balance indicate areas of concern for children with NI (Kuperminc & Stevenson 2008; Bell & Samson-Fang 2013).

There is no one perfect assessment method for dietary intake and nutrient requirements that covers all important nutritional considerations. Each method has different positive and negative aspects, which must be understood within the clinical context.

DIETARY INTAKE ASSESSMENT METHODS

Dietary intake assessment methods are used to obtain information regarding how much, how often and what types of foods and fluids an individual consumes on a regular basis. Traditionally, dietary intake assessment methods such as food records, food frequency questionnaires (FFQs) and 24-hour dietary recalls were paper-based; however, in recent years there has been an increase in the availability of electronic methods that can be accessed on a variety of mobile devices (Fuller et al. 2017). Any dietary intake assessment method relies on subjective information reported by the individual or a parent/caregiver, or a combination of both.

It is challenging to accurately assess how much a child is eating and drinking, because of variations in daily intake, reporting errors due to memory lapses for parents/carers, incorrect estimation of portion sizes consumed and reporter bias, where intake is over- or under-reported, based on what is perceived to be socially acceptable (Gibson 2005). For children with NI there are additional factors influencing reporting accuracy, including feeding problems (related to oral-pharyngeal dysphagia, and/or behavioural difficulties) or medical conditions (such as gastroesophageal reflux) that can impact dietary intake and food losses, and lead to under- or overestimations of foods and fluids consumed (Stallings et al. 1996; Kilpinen-Loisa et al. 2009; Calis et al. 2010). Furthermore, it is important to explore details regarding meal patterns, food and fluid textures managed, mealtime environments, behaviour at mealtimes, self-feeding ability, and the use of oral supplements and/or enteral feeding. These factors will not only impact on the amount of food and fluids consumed, but will influence recommendations regarding appropriate nutrition interventions. Clinicians must acknowledge dietary intake assessment may be a more complex process when working with children with NI, and devote the required time to gathering the information.

There are a variety of dietary assessment methods available to estimate intake of individuals, each with their own advantages, disadvantages and limitations (Gibson 2005). Determining absolute validity of overall dietary intake is extremely difficult; however, absolute validity for some components of dietary intake, for example energy intake, has been established in different populations (Hill & Davies 2001; Burrows et al. 2010; Walker et al. 2013). Many dietary assessment methods have established relative validity, where a test method is compared to another method, which is termed the reference method (Gibson 2005). Some methods are also more practical than others, depending on the situation. Whilst available dietary assessment methods may not be absolutely accurate, they can still provide useful information to guide management strategies.

All available methods can be grouped into two main categories – those that measure the quantity of foods and fluids consumed over a 1-day period (such as records and recalls), where the number of days assessed can be increased to obtain more accurate data on usual intakes; and those that focus more on patterns of food use during a longer time period (such as diet histories and FFQs) (Gibson 2005). Table 7.1 summarises dietary assessment methods commonly used in clinical practice, and should help clinicians determine the most appropriate method to use to obtain accurate, reliable and valid information for their client or patient.

The dietary assessment methods in Table 7.1 each have their own strengths and weak-nesses related to their intended use, ease of administration and validity. Methodologies have been used inconsistently in populations of children with NI, with little standard-isation of processes or paperwork across studies, therefore it is difficult to compare the results and hence make a 'one size fits all' recommendation. For example, one study detailed the modification of the dietary assessment method to include allowances for regurgitation, spillages, and leftover food (Walker et al. 2013); others have commented on the use of food models, the collection of brand names and food labels, and the specific instructions given to parents/carers to assist with accurate data collection (Stallings et al. 1996; Sullivan et al. 2002; Calis et al. 2010); and some have not provided any in-depth detail on the methodological procedures, limiting the reliability and applicability to clinical practice (Öztürk et al. 2004). Only one dietary assessment method (a 3-day weighed food record) has been validated via criterion standard measures in more than one population of children with NI, with mixed results (Stallings et al. 1996; Walker et al. 2013). Stallings and colleagues (1996) found significant overestimation of energy intake in a population of children with cerebral palsy (CP) aged between 2 and 18 years, concluding that the record was not a valid measure to use in clinical or research settings. On the other hand, Walker and colleagues (2013) demonstrated that a 3-day modified weighed food record accurately assessed energy intake in preschool-aged children with NI. The authors suggested that the conflicting results when compared to the Stallings (1996) study could be due to the modifications made to the record (to incorporate problems associated with feeding difficulties such as regurgitation and food and fluid spillage) as well as the increased awareness and focus of parents/carers on dietary intake in a younger cohort of children (Walker et al. 2013). The accuracy of dietary intake assessment methods in children with NI has only been established for energy intake.

Table 7.1 Summary of dietary assessment methods (Gibson 2005; Burrows et al. 2010)

Method and description	Advantages	Disadvantages	Validity for use in children with NI	Clinical utility
24-hour dietary recall				
Recall of exact intake during the previous 24 hours or preceding day (retrospective). Nutrient intake is calculated using food composition data (country-specific). Measures energy, macronutrient and micronutrient intake	• Measures actual intake • Memory aids can be used easily (e.g. food models) • Low respondent burden • Quick and inexpensive • Eating pattern less likely to be modified	• Relies on memory • One day may not be reflective of habitual intake	• No validation studies have been conducted in children with NI, hence there is no evidence that the use of 24-hour dietary recalls are accurate and reflect actual intake • Under- or over-reporting in relation to the use of the 24-hour recall in children with NI has not been examined in the literature	• Requires trained nutritionist to administer the recall • Useful in acute clinical settings when it is essential to assess actual daily intake (e.g. when a child is unwell in hospital) • Limited detail regarding contextual factors associated with eating (e.g. mealtime environment)
Repeated 24-hour dietary recall				
As above, however the recall is repeated a number of times to estimate usual food intake over a specified time period (e.g. 3 days). Measures energy, macronutrient and micronutrient intake	• As above • Measures habitual intake • Often used as a reference method against which test methods are evaluated	• Relies on memory • More time consuming than single 24-hour dietary recall	• As above	• Requires trained nutritionist to administer the recall • Useful in clinical settings to assess usual intake when other methods are deemed unsuitable (e.g. time does not allow for a full diet history to be taken)

(continued on next page)

Table 7.1 Summary of dietary assessment methods (Gibson 2005; Burrows et al. 2010) (continued)

Method and description	Advantages	Disadvantages	Validity for use in children with NI	Clinical utility
				• Limited detail regarding contextual factors associated with eating (e.g. mealtime environment) • Number, spacing and days collected to determine usual intake depends on the day-to-day variation of the nutrient of interest, which is affected by the study population and seasonal variations in intake
Weighed food record (WFR) Parent and/or child weighs all foods and fluids consumed and records intake (prospective) Measures energy, macronutrient and micronutrient intake, and can give an indication of food patterns and preferences	• Measures actual or habitual intake, depending on number of days recorded (commonly used for between 1–7 days) • Most precise method available for estimating habitual intake	• High respondent burden and time consuming • Intake may be modified due to recording • Equipment required	• Conflicting validation studies in comparison to total energy expenditure (by doubly labelled water) • Accurate for measurement of energy intake in preschool children with cerebral palsy (Walker et al. 2013)	• Parents/caregivers need training in how to complete the food record accurately • Standardised food records developed for use in typically developing children often need modification – e.g. to enable the capture of information related to spillages and regurgitation

(continued on next page)

Table 7.1 Summary of dietary assessment methods (Gibson 2005; Burrows et al. 2010) (continued)

Method and description	Advantages	Disadvantages	Validity for use in children with NI	Clinical utility
			• Overestimated energy intake by 44–54% in children with severe cerebral palsy across a broad age range (Stallings et al. 1996)	• Longer recording time frames are a greater burden to parents/caregivers and are associated with lower cooperation • Number, spacing and days collected to determine usual intake depends on the day-to-day variation of the nutrient of interest, which is affected by the study population and seasonal variations in intake
Estimated food record (EFR) Parent and/or child estimates all foods and fluids consumed (usually in household measures) and records intake (prospective) Measures energy, macronutrient and micronutrient intake, and can give an indication of food patterns and preferences	• Measures actual or habitual intake, depending on number of days recorded (commonly used for between 1–7 days)	• As above, also: • Relying on respondent to accurately estimate portion sizes	• No validation studies in children with NI • WFR and EFR are the most commonly used dietary intake assessment methods in populations of children with NI of all ages and ability levels (Stallings et al. 1996; Bergqvist et al. 2008; Kilpinen-Loisa et al. 2009; Calis et al. 2010; Walker et al. 2013)	• As above

(continued on next page)

114

Table 7.1 Summary of dietary assessment methods (Gibson 2005; Burrows et al. 2010) (continued)

Method and description	Advantages	Disadvantages	Validity for use in children with NI	Clinical utility
Measured food intake or duplicate samples				
Often used in combination with a WFR or ERF. Requires parents/caregivers to collect duplicate food samples of what is consumed by the child, which are then saved and analysed in a laboratory setting to determine nutrient intake Measures energy, macronutrient and micronutrient intake	• Measures actual or habitual intake, depending on number of days recorded	• Extremely high respondent burden and very time consuming • Extra costs associated with the production of duplicate food samples • Intake may be modified due to recording	• No validation studies in children with NI • Used to estimate dietary intake in a population of 24 children with severe cerebral palsy living in Australia. Data collected over 3 consecutive days (Schoendorfer et al. 2012)	• Not practical or recommended for use in a clinical setting or home environment because of cost, complexity, time and equipment and resources required for extensive analysis
Direct observation				
Direct observation of the foods and fluids that a child consumes over a certain time period, and recording of all details Measures energy, macronutrient and micronutrient intake, and can give an indication of food patterns and preferences depending on the number of days recorded	• Minimal burden on families if done in the home environment • Measures actual or habitual intake, depending on number of days recorded	• Cost and time associated with the use of a trained nutritionist	• Not extensively used in the literature in populations of children with NI • No validation studies have been conducted in children with NI, hence there is no evidence that the use of direct observation is accurate and reflects actual or habitual intake	• Requires trained nutritionist as observer • Need to ensure detail in recording to obtain accurate information, and consistency if using the method over time (e.g. use of specific standardised forms) • Allows observation of contextual factors impacting on mealtimes (e.g. how feeding difficulties impact intake)

(continued on next page)

Table 7.1 Summary of dietary assessment methods (Gibson 2005; Burrows et al. 2010) (continued)

Method and description	Advantages	Disadvantages	Validity for use in children with NI	Clinical utility
				• Limited practical use outside of research settings due to personnel and time requirements
Diet history (DH) Extensive interview using open-ended questions and a multiple-pass technique Measures energy, macronutrient and micronutrient intake, and food patterns and preferences	• Measures habitual intake over a longer period of time • Can be used to estimate prevalence of inadequate intakes	• Time consuming (up to 1 hour) and labour intensive • Results depend on the skill of the trained nutritionist • Relies on memory	• No validation studies have been conducted in children with NI, hence there is no evidence that the use of a DH is accurate and reflects habitual intake • Under- or over-reporting in relation to the use of the DH in children with NI has not been examined in the literature	• Requires trained nutritionist as interviewer • Can allow for qualitative data collection in regards to contextual factors that impact on dietary intake (e.g. length of meals, seating required), thus allowing for opportunities to identify areas to target when determining management strategies
Food frequency questionnaire (FFQ) Records intake over a given time frame (days to a year) using food lists, where food items are generally grouped based on their characteristics. Can be completed via	• Measures food patterns and habits, and not nutrient intake • Measures habitual diet and gives qualitative, descriptive data	• Low respondent burden • Relies on memory – may be of particular concern if looking at intake over 1 year	• Not extensively used in the literature in populations of children with NI	• Can allow for both quantitative and qualitative data collection in regards to food patterns and habits that impact on dietary intake (e.g. intake of different food groups), thus allowing for opportunities to identify areas to target when determining management strategies

(continued on next page)

Table 7.1 Summary of dietary assessment methods (Gibson 2005; Burrows et al. 2010) (continued)

Method and description	Advantages	Disadvantages	Validity for use in children with NI	Clinical utility
interview or self-administered questionnaire. Measures food patterns and food preferences			• No validation studies have been conducted in children with NI, hence there is no evidence that the use of a FFQ is accurate and reflects food patterns and habits	• Enables identification of food patterns associated with inadequate intake of specific nutrients

There have been no validation studies for macro- or micronutrient intakes in children with NI. Despite this and anecdotally, dietary intake methods can give a qualitative indication of whether a child's intake may be inadequate in particular micronutrients (e.g. low in iron if there are no significant sources of iron in the diet), prompting further investigation using objective laboratory markers if clinically indicated – for example the assessment of serum iron, transferrin, transferrin saturation and ferritin to asses iron status (Samson-Fang & Bell 2013).

The assessment of dietary intake in any population is challenging, and even more so in children with NI. Techniques suitable for controlled research environments may not be suitable for a clinical situation. The dietary assessment methods used in populations of children with NI as discussed in Table 7.1 were all performed as part of research studies, where there are often extra time and resources available to collect and interpret the dietary information. Clinicians need to consider the following details which will help guide their choice of dietary assessment method:

1. **The purpose of the dietary assessment for their client/patient.** For example, for an acutely unwell child in a hospital setting, where the purpose of the assessment is to understand the child's dietary intake within the last 24 hours, a single 24-hour dietary recall may be appropriate; alternatively, for a new client/patient to the health service where the clinician wishes to understand the child's usual dietary intake and what factors impact this, a diet history may be the method of choice.

2. **The setting where the dietary assessment will take place.** For example, in a clinical outpatient setting, an inpatient setting or in the home environment.

3. **The ability of the parent/caregiver to participate – balancing burden with accurate information.** For example, the accuracy of dietary information may be compromised if a parent/caregiver is given a long, time-consuming weighed food record to complete when the clinician is aware that the family has a very busy schedule. This may also weaken the relationship between the parent/caregiver and clinician. Family-specific factors need to be considered when choosing a dietary assessment method.

4. **The context and mealtime environment.** Obtaining qualitative information about the context and other factors influencing dietary intake is just as important as the quantifiable dietary intake data for successful, patient-centred, long-term nutritional management of children with NI.

NUTRITIONAL REQUIREMENTS

Despite the common nature of nutritional challenges in children with NI, there is very little evidence available regarding particular nutritional requirements. Many clinicians, therefore, are unsure how to most accurately estimate the nutritional requirements in this population to ensure optimal weight gain and growth.

Energy Requirements

The energy requirements of individuals are best determined through the measurement of total energy expenditure (TEE) – this refers to the amount of energy (or calories) that the body needs each day to carry out its usual functions (FAO/WHO/UNU 2001). The three components of TEE include (1) the resting energy expenditure, which is a combination of basal metabolic rate (BMR, the amount of energy required by your body to perform vital functions such as breathing) and the energy cost of arousal, and contributes between 60–75% of TEE; (2) diet-induced thermogenesis, which is the energy required to digest, absorb and transport nutrients, and makes up approximately 10% of TEE; and (3) the energy expended during physical activity (Poehlman 1989).

The energy requirements for children with NI differ from current recommendations for typically developing children (TDC), and depend on a number of factors which can influence TEE. These factors are described below:

- **Type and severity of NI** – this can influence patterns of movement and muscle function, which then alter the amount of energy a child uses per day, hence impacting energy requirements (Rieken et al. 2011; Walker et al. 2012).

- **Differences in body composition** – muscle tissue is more metabolically active when compared to body fat, therefore the amount and proportion of each of these tissues will influence how much energy a child requires (Bandini et al. 1991; Bell & Davies 2010; Walker et al. 2012).

- **Altered growth patterns** – children with NI may be shorter and lighter than their typically developing peers, which will mean that their energy requirement will be different (van den Berg Emons et al. 1995; Bell & Davies 2010).

- **Physical activity levels** – the amount of physical activity performed each day greatly impacts energy requirements. A child with NI, therefore, who is non-ambulant and has lower physical activity levels, will generally have a lower energy requirement when compared to an ambulant TDC of the same age, sex, body composition and weight (Bandini et al. 1991; Stallings et al. 1996; Walker et al. 2012). Physical activity levels for individuals with NI may be due to voluntary and involuntary movements (Johnson et al. 1997).

The majority of literature which describes the measurement of TEE in children with NI demonstrates that at a population level, energy requirements for children with NI are significantly lower when compared to age- and sex-matched TDC, due to lower amounts of fat-free mass and lower physical activity levels (Bandini et al. 1995; van den Berg Emons et al. 1995, Stallings et al. 1996; Bell & Davies 2010; Walker et al. 2012). Studies have shown that this difference can be quite significant, with energy requirements for children with NI who are non-ambulant up to 30–40% lower than TDC (Stallings et al.

1996; Vernon-Roberts et al. 2010; Walker et al. 2012). Particular research findings that are of interest and should be considered include:

- Children with spasticity had decreased energy requirements when compared to TDC due to reduced physical activity levels and decreased resting energy expenditure (Bandini et al. 1991; van den Berg Emons et al. 1995; Stallings et al. 1996; Bell & Davies 2010; Walker et al. 2012).

- A lower energy requirement has been observed in children who are fed via gastrostomy when compared to those who are orally fed (Sullivan et al. 2006; Rieken et al. 2011). This is possibly due to the increased severity of gross motor impairment and resultant lower levels of physical activity of those who are gastrostomy fed.

- Children with NI who were ambulant and had similar body compositions to TDC also had similar energy requirements to TDC (Bell & Davies 2010; Walker et al. 2012).

- Adult studies have demonstrated an increased energy requirement for those with dyskinesia compared to adults with spasticity due to involuntary movement patterns (Johnson et al. 1996, 1997). It has been hypothesised that children with NI with dyskinetic movement disorders will have similar or even increased energy requirements when compared to TDC as a result of involuntary movements at rest that increase physical activity levels.

Estimating Energy Requirements in the Clinical Setting

Because of the associated high costs, increased burden on children, families and researchers/clinicians, and extensive time involved, measurement of total energy expenditure is limited to research settings. To determine the energy requirements of children with NI in the clinical setting, estimation equations must be utilised. Because of the complexities and heterogeneity of NI, estimating energy requirements for this group is not straightforward. There are no adequately validated population-specific equations suitable for this purpose.

Two population-specific equations have been described in the literature (Krick et al. 1992; Rieken et al. 2011). The first was developed from a retrospective audit of the medical records of 32 children with CP aged between 9 months and 18 years, most of whom were non-ambulant (Krick et al. 1992). It was later compared to measured total energy expenditure via the doubly labelled water method, and was proven to be inaccurate (Rieken et al. 2011). In 2011, Rieken and colleagues developed two equations based on measured total energy expenditure (via doubly labelled water) and body composition of 52 children with CP aged between 2 and 19 years, all of whom were non-ambulant. Both equations have been shown to be inaccurate, underestimating energy requirements by approximately 22% when compared to total energy expenditure measured via doubly labelled water in 11 children with CP aged between 2.9 and 4.4 years, all of whom were non-ambulant (Walker et al. 2012). These equations, therefore, are currently not recommended for use in clinical practice.

Recent consensus guidelines from the European Society of Paediatric Gastroenterology, Hepatology and Nutrition recommend using dietary reference standards for TDC to estimate energy requirements for children with NI, with particular reference to the Schofield equations (Romano et al. 2017). The Schofield equations (Schofield 1985) are simple and easy to use, and require only a measure of body weight to estimate basal metabolic rate. An estimation of physical activity levels is then required to calculate energy requirements. The equations are detailed in Table 7.2. International recommendations for multiples of BMR for TDC range from 1.3 to 2.15 depending on age and physical activity level (FAO/WHO/UNU 2001).

Table 7.2 Schofield prediction equations commonly used in paediatric populations to estimate energy requirements (Schofield 1985)

Schofield prediction equations to estimate basal metabolic rate in MJ/day
0–3 years
Males: (0.249 x weight) – 0.127
Females: (0.244 x weight) – 0.130
3–10 years
Males: (0.095 x weight) + 2.110
Females: (0.085 x weight) + 2.033
10–18 years
Males: (0.074 x weight) + 2.754
Females: (0.056 x weight) + 2.898

Comments pertaining to the equations

- The equations only require a child's weight as a measured variable
- The equations displayed estimate an individual's BMR – the clinician is then required to multiply the BMR by an appropriate physical activity level to obtain an estimated energy requirement
- International recommendations for physical activity levels for TDC range from 1.3 to 2.15 depending on age and sex (FAO/WHO/UNU 2001)
- Recommended physical activity levels for children with NI who are more severely impaired differ from those for TDC, and the following values should be used:
  - Wheelchair dependent (Gross Motor Function Classification System [GMFCS] III–V) – 1.1 to 1.2 (Stallings et al. 1996)
  - Non-wheelchair dependent (GMFCS I and II) – 1.6 (Bell & Davies 2010)
  - Wheelchair dependent with significant involuntary movements 1.6 to 1.8 (Johnson et al. 1996, 1997)

Recommendations and practical considerations for estimating energy requirements in clinical practice

1. In the absence of accurate, population-specific prediction equations, clinicians should use prediction equations developed for use in TDC, but with caution
   - The equations are a starting point on which to base recommendations for dietary intakes as they only give an indication of energy requirements
   - Energy requirements for children with NI are frequently less than those of TDC

2. Energy requirements need to be individualised, and clinicians need to understand the impact of the type and severity of NI, body composition levels, altered growth patterns and physical activity levels on estimated energy requirements, and use clinical judgement

3. Recommendations for nutrition interventions based on estimated energy requirements must be combined with regular monitoring, assessment and evaluation of dietary intake, growth (in particular, weight gain) and nutritional status over time to ensure optimal growth and development

The Schofield equations were developed from healthy, typical populations of adults and children involving over 100 separate studies (Schofield 1985). These equations have been shown to give inconsistent results for children with NI and caution must be exercised with their use (Bandini et al. 1991; Azcue et al. 1996; Stallings et al. 1996; Hogan 2004; Walker et al. 2012). Given the inaccuracy of any method to estimate energy requirements of children with NI, these formulae are a starting point only. Regular monitoring and follow-up is essential to ensure that the desired level of positive energy balance is achieved but not exceeded for appropriate growth and development. The most sensitive indicator of energy balance is body weight, with longer-term outcomes including measurement of body composition also helpful.

Macronutrient Requirements

The majority of literature regarding nutritional requirements in children with NI has focused on energy requirements. When examining the literature in relation to macronutrients, most studies in populations of children with NI report intakes in relation to body composition for a particular age group, compared to a group of TDC, or compared to national recommendations, rather than actually investigating requirements (Sullivan et al. 2002; Walker et al. 2012). Macronutrient intake contributes to overall energy intake, and is essential for optimal growth and development in all children. Lower energy requirements therefore will result in lower overall macronutrient intakes.

There is currently no evidence-base to support the idea that children with NI have altered macronutrient requirements when compared to TDC. Clinicians, therefore, should aim to achieve national country-specific or international (FAO/WHO 1997; FAO/WHO/ UNU 2007; FAO 2010) recommendations for macronutrient requirements for TDC, whilst using clinical judgement to ensure optimal intake.

Carbohydrate Requirements

Carbohydrates provide the major energy source for the body, and are an important part of daily dietary intake for all children (FAO/WHO 1997). Carbohydrates should generally provide between 45–65% of daily total energy intake (FAO/WHO 1997). Intake of carbohydrates in groups of children with NI have been detailed in the literature, and generally fall within the recommended percentage intake; however it is overall energy intake that is often reduced (Grammatikopoulou et al. 2009; Kilpinen-Loisa et al. 2009).

Protein Requirements

Protein is an important macronutrient that is used in the body to help build new cells and repair tissues, and is an important component of enzymes and hormones (FAO/WHO/UNU 2007). It is required for adequate growth and development in all children, in particular contributing to lean muscle tissue gain. Studies in populations of children with NI have demonstrated lower intakes of protein when compared to age- and sex-matched TDC, most probably attributable to a lower energy intake (Walker et al. 2012).

There is currently no evidence to suggest that the protein requirements for children with NI differ to that of TDC. It is recommended, therefore, that country-specific or FAO/ WHO/UNU (2007) nutrient reference values are used to determine protein requirements according to age and sex using the grams of protein per kilogram of body weight method (see Table 7.3). Because of the lower energy requirements of some children with NI a higher intake of protein as a percentage of energy intake may be required when compared to recommendations, to ensure adequate growth and development. Children with NI who are undernourished may require additional protein intake to promote catch-up growth. Recommendations once again are similar to that for TDC – an intake of 2.0g/kg/day of protein combined with an increase of energy intake by 20% (Bell & Samson-Fang 2013).

Fat Requirements

Fat provides the greatest amount of energy at 37kJ (or 9 calories) per gram, and should account for between 20% and 35% of total daily energy intake. This will ensure that fat-soluble vitamin intake is optimised, and will sustain body weight (FAO 2010). Fat is

Table 7.3 International recommended intakes for protein for typically developing children (FAO/WHO/UNU 2007)

Age	Protein intake (g/kg/day)
3–6 months	1.85
6–9 months	1.65
9–12 months	1.50
1–2 years	1.20
2–3 years	1.15
3–5 years	1.10
5–12 years	1.00
Boys	
12–14 years	1.0
14–16 years	0.95
16–18 years	0.90
Girls	
12–14 years	0.95
14–16 years	0.90
16–18 years	0.80

an essential part of the diet and is important for good health. Supplementation of fats is often used as part of nutritional management strategies to help increase overall energy intake in children with NI who may be struggling to maintain their weight. Clinicians must be careful in their nutritional management for children with NI, and achieve a balance between protein and fat intake when increasing energy intake. An inappropriate increase in fat intake in the diet, whilst promoting weight gain and growth, can also lead to the excessive deposition of fat in children with NI, putting them at increased risk of developing overweight and obesity and associated complications (Sullivan et al. 2006; Vernon-Roberts et al. 2010).

Micronutrient Requirements

As is the case with macronutrient requirements, literature regarding specific micronutrient requirements for children with NI is lacking. Micronutrient intakes of children with NI are often less than those of TDC (Sullivan et al. 2002; Kalra et al. 2015) and children with NI are more likely to have clinical micronutrient deficiencies (Papadopoulos et al. 2008; Kalra et al. 2015). Recommendations for micronutrient intakes of children with NI should be based on dietary reference values for TDC, which can be viewed in Table 7.4 and Table 7.5 (Romano et al. 2017).

Table 7.4 International recommended mineral intakes for typically developing children (FAO/WHO 2001)

Group	Calcium (mg/day)	Selenium (µg/day)	Magnesium (mg/day)	Zinc[a] (mg/day)	Iron[b] (mg/day)	Iodine (µg/day)
Infants						
0–6 months	300[c]–400[d]	6	26[c]–36[e]	2.8	[f]	90
7–12 months	400	10	54	4.1	6.2–18.6	90
Children						
1–3 years	500	17	60	4.1	3.9–11.6	90
4–6 years	600	22	76	4.8	4.2–12.6	90
7–9 years	700	21	100	5.6	5.9–17.8	120 (6–12 yrs)
Adolescents						
Females						
10–18 years	1300	26	220	7.2	9.3–28.0 (11–14 yrs, pre-menarche) 21.8–65.4 (11–14 yrs) 20.7–62.0 (15–17 yrs)	150 (13–18 yrs)
Males						
10–18 years	1300	32	230	8.6	9.7–29.2 (11–14 yrs) 12.5–37.6 (15–17 yrs)	150 (13–18 yrs)

[a]Assuming moderate bioavailability
[b]Range detailed from low (5%) to high (15%) bioavailability
[c]Breastfed
[d]Cow milk-fed
[e]Formula-fed
[f]Neonatal iron stores are sufficient to meet the iron requirement for the first 6 months in term infants

Table 7.5 International recommended vitamin intakes for typically developing children (FAO/WHO 2001)

Group	Vit C (mg/d)	Thiamine (mg/d)	Riboflavin (mg/d)	Niacin (mg NE/d)[a]	Vit B6 (mg/d)	Pantothenate (mg/d)	Biotin (µg/d)	Vit B12 (µg/d)	Folate (µg RE/d)[b]	Vit A (µg RE/d)[c]	Vit D (µg/d)	Vit E (mg α-TE/d)[d]	Vit K (µg/d)
Infants													
0–6 months	25	0.2	0.3	2	0.1	1.7	5	0.4	80	375	5	2.7	5[e]
7–12 months	30	0.3	0.4	4	0.3	1.8	6	0.7	80	400	5	2.7	10
Children													
1–3 years	30	0.5	0.5	6	0.5	2.0	8	0.9	150	400	5	5.0	15
4–6 years	30	0.6	0.6	8	0.6	3.0	12	1.2	200	450	5	5.0	20
7–9 years	35	0.9	0.9	12	1.0	4.0	20	1.8	300	500	5	7.0	25
Adolescents													
Females													
10–18 years	40	1.1	1.0	16	1.2	5.0	25	2.4	400	600	5	7.5	35–55
Males													
10–18 years	40	1.2	1.3	16	1.3	5.0	25	2.4	400	600	5	10.0	35–55

[a]NE = niacin equivalents
[b]DFE = dietary folate equivalents
[c]Vitamin A values are 'recommended safe intakes' instead of recommended vitamin intakes
[d]Data were not strong enough to formulate recommendations. Figures represent the best estimate of requirements. TE = tocopherol equivalents
[e]This intake cannot be met by infants who are exclusively breast-fed. All breast-fed infants should receive vitamin K supplementation at birth according to nationally approved guidelines

Children with NI who have a low energy intake often have challenges meeting their micronutrient requirements, and may require supplementation in addition to their usual intake (Bell & Samson-Fang 2013). Vitamin D and calcium intakes are of particular importance for children with NI, because of the relationship with bone health (Kuperminc & Stevenson 2008). Starting doses of between 800 and 1000IU of vitamin D in those children at risk of osteoporosis (those who are wheelchair dependent with limited sunlight exposure or children on long-term anticonvulsants) should be considered (Ozel et al. 2016). Further, vitamin D status should be monitored and additional supplementation should be considered if levels are insufficient (Fehlings et al. 2012; Ozel et al. 2016). Children with NI are at greater risk of iron deficiency due to low iron intakes (Sullivan et al. 2002).

Fluid Requirements

Water is an essential nutrient required for many bodily processes, including the digestion, absorption and transportation of nutrients, among other functions. The fluid requirements for children with NI are similar to and should be based on those for TDC – there is no evidence to suggest otherwise (Romano et al. 2017). It can, however, be difficult for many children with NI to achieve an adequate fluid intake, because of factors such as feeding and swallowing difficulties, poor feed tolerance (which may result in frequent fluid loss via regurgitation and vomiting), increased losses via saliva, and an inability to effectively communicate thirst. Therefore, particular attention must be paid to hydration status in those children who may be more susceptible to an inadequate intake. It is important to ensure regular review of both dietary intake and nutritional status, including looking for signs of dehydration (and assisting parents/carers to be able to monitor and identify this as well). Dry, cracked lips and/or a dry mouth, a decreased urine output, darker-coloured urine, drowsiness or irritability which is out of the ordinary, sunken eyes or dizziness or light-headedness can all potentially indicate that a child is not receiving enough fluids.

SUMMARY

The assessment of dietary intake in children with NI is a critical part of the overall nutritional management. Whilst it can often be challenging, the use of clinical judgement combined with frequent monitoring can help ensure optimal growth and development for children with NI. The following key practice points are relevant in all clinical settings:

- There is no one method that will accurately assess dietary intake in children with NI. All methods give an estimate of dietary intake, and the choice of method will depend on the purpose of the dietary intake assessment, the setting in which the assessment is conducted, and the ability of the parents/carers to be involved. Often a combination of both quantitative and qualitative data including nutrient intake, food habits and preferences and context-specific information (such as mealtime environments) can be best to inform comprehensive management strategies.

- The energy requirements of children with NI can differ from TDC, and are generally lower. However, in the absence of any validated equations to estimate energy requirements in children with NI, clinicians should base their estimations on requirements for TDC, and adjust as required. Overestimation of energy needs can lead to excessive deposition of body fat, and an increased risk of overweight and obesity (Sullivan et al. 2006; Vernon-Roberts et al. 2010).

- Similarly, macronutrient and micronutrient requirements for children with NI should be based on those for TDC, and adjusted as required.

- Appropriate positive energy balance, as evidenced by adequate weight gain and growth, is a common clinical indicator used to determine if a child with NI is meeting their energy requirements.

- Children with NI can have difficulty achieving an adequate fluid intake, so an increased focus on fluid intake for susceptible children is essential. Fluid requirements should be based on recommendations for TDC and adjusted as required.

REFERENCES

Azcue MP, Zello GA, Levy LD, Pencharz PB (1996) Energy expenditure and body composition in children with spastic quadriplegic cerebral palsy. *J Pediatr* 129: 870–876.

Bandini LG, Schoeller DA, Fukagawa NK, Wykes LJ, Dietz WH (1991) Body composition and energy expenditure in adolescents with cerebral palsy or myelodysplasia. *Pediatr Res* 29: 70–77.

Bandini LG, Puelzl Quinn H, Morelli JA Fukagawa NK (1995) Estimation of energy requirements in persons with severe central nervous system impairment. *J Pediatr* 126: 828–832.

Bell KL, Davies PS (2010) Energy expenditure and physical activity of ambulatory children with cerebral palsy and of typically developing children. *Am J Clin Nutr* 92: 313–319.

Bell KL, Samson-Fang L (2013) Nutritional management of children with cerebral palsy. *Eur J Clin Nutr* 67(Suppl 2): S13–16.

Bergqvist AG, Trabulsi J, Schall JI, Stallings, VA (2008) Growth failure in children with intractable epilepsy is not due to increased resting energy expenditure. *Dev Med Child Neurol* 50: 439–444.

Brooks J, Day S, Shavelle R, Strauss D (2011) Low weight, morbidity, and mortality in children with cerebral palsy: new clinical growth charts. *Pediatrics* 128: e299–307.

Burrows TL, Martin RJ, Collins CE (2010) A systematic review of the validity of dietary assessment methods in children when compared with the method of doubly labeled water. *J Am Diet Assoc* 110: 1501–1510.

Calis EaC, Veugelers R, Rieken R, Tibboel D, Evenhuis HM, Penning C (2010) Energy intake does not correlate with nutritional status in children with severe generalised cerebral palsy and intellectual disability. *Clin Nutr* 29: 617–621.

FAO (2010) *Fats and Fatty Acids in Human Nutrition: Report of an Expert Consultation*. Geneva: World Health Organization.

FAO/WHO (1997) *Carbohydrates in Human Nutrition: Report of a Joint FAO/WHO Expert Consultation*. Rome: FAO/WHO.

FAO/WHO (2001) *Human Vitamin and Mineral Requirements: Report of a Joint FAO/WHO Expert Consultation*. Bangkok: FAO/WHO.

FAO/WHO/UNU (2001) *Human Energy Requirements: Report of a Joint FAO/WHO/UNU Expert Consultation. Food and Nutrition Technical Report Series 1*. Rome: FAO/WHO/UNU.

FAO/WHO/UNU (2007) *Protein and Amino Acid Requirements in Human Nutrition: Report of a Joint FAO/WHO/UNU Expert Consultation. WHO Technical Report Series 935*. FAO/WHO/UNU.

Fehlings D, Switzer L, Agarwal P et al. (2012) Informing evidence-based clinical practice guidelines for children with cerebral palsy at risk of osteoporosis: a systematic review. *Dev Med Child Neurol* 54: 106–116.

Fuller NR, Fong M, Gerofi J et al. (2017) Comparison of an electronic versus traditional food diary for assessing dietary intake – a validation study. *Obes Res Clin Pract* 11: 647–654.

Gibson R (2005) *Principles of Nutritional Assessment*. New York: Oxford University Press.

Grammatikopoulou MG, Daskalou E, Tsigga M (2009) Diet, feeding practices, and anthropometry of children and adolescents with cerebral palsy and their siblings. *Nutrition* 25: 620–626.

Hill RJ, Davies PSW (2001) The validity of self reported energy intake as determined by the doubly labelled water technique. *Br J Nutr* 85: 415–430.

Hogan SE (2004) Energy requirements of children with cerebral palsy. *Can J Diet Pract Res* 65: 124–130.

Johnson RK, Goran MI, Ferrara MS, Poehlman ET (1996) Athetosis increases resting metabolic rate in adults with cerebral palsy. *J Am Diet Assoc* 96: 145–148.

Johnson RK, Hildreth HG, Contompasis SH, Goran MI (1997) Total energy expenditure in adults with cerebral palsy as assessed by doubly labeled water. *J Am Diet Assoc* 97: 966–970.

Kalra S, Aggarwal A, Chillar N, Faridi MM (2015) Comparison of micronutrient levels in children with cerebral palsy and neurologically normal controls. *Indian J Pediatr* 82: 140–144.

Kilpinen-Loisa P, Pihko H, Vesander U, Paganus A, Ritanen U, Makitie O (2009) Insufficient energy and nutrient intake in children with motor disability. *Acta Paediatrica* 98: 1329–1333.

Krick J, Murphy PE, Markham JF, Shapiro BK (1992) A proposed formula for calculating energy needs of children with cerebral palsy. *Dev Med Child Neurol* 34: 481–487.

Kuperminc MN, Stevenson RD (2008) Growth and nutrition disorders in children with cerebral palsy. *Dev Disabil Res Rev* 14: 137–146.

Oftedal S, Davies PS, Boyd RN et al. (2017) Body composition, diet, and physical activity: a longitudinal cohort study in preschoolers with cerebral palsy. *Am J Clin Nutr* 105: 369–378.

Ozel S, Switzer L, Macintosh A, Fehlings D (2016) Informing evidence-based clinical practice guidelines for children with cerebral palsy at risk of osteoporosis: an update. *Dev Med Child Neurol* 58: 918–923.

Öztürk M, Kutluhan S, Demirci S et al. (2004) Dietary assessment of children with cerebral palsy: case control study in Isparta. *Eur J Med* 9: 22–25.

Papadopoulos A, Ntaios G, Kaiafa G et al. (2008) Increased incidence of iron deficiency anemia secondary to inadequate iron intake in institutionalized, young patients with cerebral palsy. *Int J Hematol* 88: 495–497.

Poehlman ET (1989) A review: exercise and its influence on resting energy metabolism in man. *Med Sci Sports Exerc* 21: 515–525.

Rieken R, Van Goudoever JB, Schierbeek H et al. (2011) Measuring body composition and energy expenditure in children with severe neurologic impairment and intellectual disability. *Am J Clin Nutr* 94: 759–766.

Romano C, Van Wynckel M, Hulst J et al. (2017) European Society for Paediatric Gastroenterology, Hepatology and Nutrition guidelines for the evaluation and treatment of gastrointestinal and nutritional complications in children with neurological impairment. *J Pediatr Gastroent Nutr* 65: 242–264.

Samson-Fang L, Bell KL (2013) Assessment of growth and nutrition in children with cerebral palsy. *Eur J Clin Nutr* 67(Suppl 2): S5–8.

Schoendorfer N, Tinggi U, Sharp N, Boyd R, Vitetta L, Davies PS (2012) Protein levels in enteral feeds: do these meet requirements in children with severe cerebral palsy? *Br J Nutr* 107: 1476–1481.

Schofield WN (1985) Predicting basal metabolic rate, new standards and review of previous work. *Hum Nutr Clin Nutr* 39C: S5–41.

Stallings VA, Zemel BS, Davies JC, Cronk CE, Charney EB (1996) Energy expenditure of children and adolescents with severe disabilities: a cerebral palsy model. *Am J Clin Nutr* 64: 627–34.

Stevenson RD, Conaway M, Chumlea W et al. (2006) Growth and health in children with moderate-to-severe cerebral palsy. *Pediatrics* 118: 1010–1018.

Sullivan PB, Juszczak E, Lambert BR, Rose M, Ford-Adams ME, Johnson A (2002) Impact of feeding problems on nutritional intake and growth: Oxford Feeding Study II. *Dev Med Child Neurol* 44: 461–467.

Sullivan PB, Alder N, Bachlet A et al. (2006) Gastrostomy feeding in cerebral palsy: too much of a good thing? *Dev Med Child Neurol* 48(11): 877–882.

van den Berg Emons HJ, Saris WH, De Barbanson DC, Westerterp KR, Huson A, Van Baak MA (1995) Daily physical activity of school children with spastic diplegia and of healthy control subjects. *J Pediatr* 127: 578–584.

Vernon-Roberts A, Wells J, Grant H et al. (2010) Gastrostomy feeding in cerebral palsy: enough and no more. *Dev Med Child Neurol* 52: 1099–1105.

Walker JL, Bell KL, Boyd RN, Davies PS (2012) Energy requirements in preschool-age children with cerebral palsy. *Am J Clin Nutr* 96: 1309–1315.

Walker JL, Bell KL, Boyd RN, Davies PS (2013) Validation of a modified three-day weighed food record for measuring energy intake in preschool-aged children with cerebral palsy. *Clin Nutr* 32: 426–431.

CHAPTER 8

Assessment of Nutritional State: Micronutrient Deficiencies and Bone Health

Heidi H Kecskemethy and Steven J Bachrach

INTRODUCTION

Bone health is complex and is related to intrinsic (genetic, ethnicity, sex, age, family history) and extrinsic (nutritional intake/status, activity level, smoking, body weight, medication use, alcohol consumption) factors. In patients with neurological conditions, particular attention should be directed to the extrinsic factors, which might be controlled to decrease risk to bone health. The focus of this chapter is on a key extrinsic factor in bone health-nutrition. Also in this chapter, a summary of bone assessment and treatment interventions will be provided.

DIET/NUTRITION

Diet plays an important role in bone health for all populations. Nutritional status is directly related to bone health in patients with neuromuscular conditions. Compromised nutrition is associated with growth deficiency and lack of bone mineral accrual in growing bones, and in lower bone mineral density (BMD) and fracture across all ages (Henderson et al. 2002, 2004; Händel et al. 2015; Mazidi et al. 2018).

Nutrients of Concern for Bone Health

The two most important nutrients for bone health are calcium and vitamin D. Calcium is a major component of bone tissue, and the skeleton serves as the largest calcium reservoir in the body. Bones store 99% of the body's calcium. Calcium is not made in the body – it must be ingested and absorbed. Vitamin D ensures effective absorption of dietary calcium; lack of adequate vitamin D negatively impacts calcium absorption.

In addition to bone and tooth formation, calcium is used for other physiological functions such as muscle contractions, nerve impulse transmission, heartbeat regulation, regulation of blood pressure, and other critical physiological processes. If the body has inadequate dietary calcium, calcium is removed from where it is stored in bones and is used for more essential functions. Over time, this can weaken bones, leading to undermineralised, fragile bones that break easily (osteoporosis) (Beto 2015).

Vitamin D deficiency in children leads to rickets, which causes bone weakness, bowed legs and other skeletal deformities, such as stooped posture. In adults, very low vitamin D levels can result in osteomalacia (soft bone), causing bone pain and deformities of the long bones. In both conditions, the risk for fractures is increased.

Several other nutrients that contribute to bone health include phosphorus, magnesium, zinc and vitamins C and K (Table 8.1).

Reference Standards

Recommended intake levels for macro- and micronutrients vary worldwide. The World Health Organization and Food and Agricultural Organization of the United Nations are organisations that are involved worldwide with health and nutrition. These organisations work with health ministries and similar entities within countries and regions of the world to help establish nutrition standards and nutrient recommendations. Below are some example reference standards.

The European Food Safety Authority reviews and updates reference values for nutrient and energy intakes for the European Union. Dietary Reference Values for the EU can be found here:

https://www.efsa.europa.eu/sites/default/files/assets/DRV_Summary_tables_jan_17.pdf

The Food and Nutrition Board of the Institute of Medicine, National Academy of Sciences establishes Dietary Reference Intakes for macro- and micronutrients for the USA. Dietary Reference Intakes for nutrients can be found here:

https://ods.od.nih.gov/Health_Information/Dietary_Reference_Intakes.aspx

Table 8.1 Nutrients of concern for bone health

Nutrient	Function	Sign of deficiency	Food sources
Calcium	• Builds and maintains bones and teeth • Essential in blood clotting • Influences transmission of ions across cell membranes • Required in nerve transmission	• Rickets – abnormal development of bones • Low bone mineral density, and eventually fractures	Dairy: yoghurt, cheese, milk Grains: fortified or enriched grain products Vegetables: green leafy vegetables (such as collards, kale, mustard greens and turnip greens) Other: fortified beverages, tofu made with calcium sulfate Meat/Fish/Eggs: sardines, salmon
Vitamin D	• Necessary for the formation of normal bone • Promotes the absorption of calcium and phosphorus in the intestines	• Rickets in children, osteomalacia in adults • Fractures	Dairy: fortified milk and products (North America) Meat/Fish/Eggs: egg yolk, liver, fatty fish
Phosphorus	• Builds and maintains bones and teeth • Component of nucleic acids, phospholipids • Coenzyme functions in energy metabolism • Buffers intracellular fluid	• Phosphate depletion unusual • Affects renal, neuromuscular, skeletal systems and blood chemistries	Dairy: cheese Grains: whole-grain breads, cereals and other grain products Meat/Fish/Eggs: egg yolk, meat, poultry, fish Other: legumes
Magnesium	• Required for many coenzyme oxidation–phosphorylation reactions, nerve impulse transmissions, and for muscle contraction	• Muscular hyperexcitability (tremors, convulsions, irritability, tetany) • Fatigue • Loss of appetite • Apathy, confusion • Sound and light sensitivity • Anxiety • Insomnia • Irritability	Grains: whole-grain breads, cereals and other grain products Vegetables: green vegetables Other: tofu, legumes

(continued on next page)

133

Table 8.1 Nutrients of concern for bone health (Continued)

Nutrient	Function	Sign of deficiency	Food sources
Zinc	• Component of many enzyme systems and insulin	• Decreased wound healing • Hypogonadism • Mild anaemia • Decreased taste • Hair loss • Diarrhoea • Growth failure • Skin changes	Grains: whole-grain breads, cereals and other fortified or enriched grain products Meat/Fish/Eggs: meat, liver, egg yolk, oysters and other seafood Other: legumes
Vitamin C	• Essential in: synthesis of collagen and iron absorption and transport • Antioxidant • Functions in folate metabolism	• Scurvy • Petechiae • Bleeding gums • Osmotic diarrhoea	Fruit: citrus, papaya, cantaloupe, berries Vegetables: potatoes, cabbage
Vitamin K	• Catalyses prothrombin synthesis, required in the synthesis of other blood clotting factors	• Prolonged bleeding and prothrombin time • Haemorrhagic manifestations (especially in newborn infants)	Vegetables: green leafy vegetables Meat/Fish/Eggs: pork, liver Fats: vegetable oils

Dietary Reference Intakes for Canada were established in conjunction with Health Canada and the Institute of Medicine. Current recommendations can be found here:

https://www.canada.ca/en/health-canada/services/food-nutrition/healthy-eating/dietary-reference-intakes.html

New Zealand and Australia utilise a version of the Canadian reference values:

https://www.nrv.gov.au/nutrients

Vitamin D Deficiency and its Relation to Bone Health
The Physiological Role of Vitamin D

Vitamin D is a pro-hormone that is essential for absorption of calcium from the gastro-intestinal tract. Sources of vitamin D are skin exposure to sunlight and dietary ingestion of vitamin D in food and supplements.

In the dermis and epidermis, ultraviolet B radiation converts 7-dehydrocholesterol to vitamin D3. Dietary or supplementary vitamin D (which can be D2 or D3) as well as vitamin D3 from the skin undergoes hydroxylation in the liver (to 25-hydroxy-vitamin D) and again in the kidney (to 1,25-dihydroxy-vitamin D or calcitriol). The renal hydroxylation of vitamin D is tightly regulated, and is stimulated by parathyroid hormone (PTH), hypocalcaemia and hypophosphataemia. The major role of calcitriol is to maintain serum calcium and phosphorus levels in a physiological range. It does so by increasing absorption of calcium and phosphorus from the gastrointestinal tract, increasing renal tubular reabsorption of calcium, and mobilising calcium and phosphorus from the skeleton. The half-life of 25-OH-vitD is 2–3 weeks, compared to only 4 hours for 1,25-dihydroxy-vitD. 25-OH-vitD is the major circulating form of vitamin D (levels are 1000 times that of 1,25-dihydroxy-vitD). For these reasons, levels of 25-OH-vitD are the best indicator of total body vitamin D status. The kidney can also metabolise 25-OH-vitD to an inactive metabolite (24,25-dihydroxy-vitD). This metabolic pathway is enhanced by two frequently used anticonvulsants, phenobarbital and phenytoin, resulting in lower levels of 25-OH-vitD.

Serum vitamin D levels within populations are affected by a combination of dietary practices and intake (food supply fortification with vitamin D practices vary around the world) as well as sun exposure. Recommendations for sun avoidance, including use of sunblock, lifestyle choices involving indoor activities, degree of skin pigmentation and style of dress may place much of the population at risk for low or insufficient serum levels of vitamin D. Studies from the UK have estimated that approximately 9 minutes of daily sun exposure (including forearms and legs) at lunchtime from March to September for white Caucasians and 25 minutes for those with highly pigmented skin is enough to

Table 8.2 Classification of serum 25-OH-vitamin D levels

Institute of Medicine (IOM 2010)	The Endocrine Society (Holick et al. 2011)	Status
< 12	< 20	Deficient
12–19	20–29	Insufficient
20–50	30–50	Sufficient
> 50	> 50	High

maintain sufficient vitamin D levels throughout the winter (Webb et al. 2018a, 2018b). It was estimated in another study that exposure time in the southern USA to achieve one minimum erythema dose is 4–10 minutes for pale skin and 60–80 minutes for dark skin (Holick 2004). Thus for many people, especially those with highly pigmented skin, ingestion of vitamin D is necessary to achieve sufficient levels.

CLASSIFICATION OF SERUM VITAMIN D LEVELS

Serum 25-OH-vitamin D results are classified into levels: deficient, insufficient, sufficient and high. Currently, there are two differing recommendations for the classification of serum 25-OH-vitamin D levels (Table 8.2).

VITAMIN D DEFICIENCY

Vitamin D deficiency in the general population is quite common, as evidenced by studies from around the world (Priemel et al. 2010; Hoge et al. 2015; Manios et al. 2017; Liu et al. 2018). This chapter will not be discussing non-nutritional rickets, such as those caused by genetic mutations (X-linked hypophosphataemia) or severe liver or kidney disease.

In a vitamin D deficient state, intestinal calcium absorption is only 10–15% (instead of 30–60% when vitamin D levels are sufficient) (Misra et al. 2008). This stimulates the production of PTH, which helps maintain a normal serum calcium at the expense of the bones, the main calcium stores. An increased PTH level also causes phosphorus losses in urine. Decreased levels of phosphorus and calcium cause decreased bone mineralisation.

Failure of mineralisation of osteoid leads to rickets in growing/immature bones and to osteomalacia in mature bones. The low phosphorus levels cause a failure of expected apoptosis of hypertrophied chondrocytes, with resulting disorganisation of the growth plate. Failure or delay of mineralisation of osteoid, as well as abnormal organisation of the growth plate and impairment of cartilage mineralisation, are the hallmarks of the pathology of rickets. This leads to the classic findings on X-ray, including metaphyseal widening and fraying, cortical thinning of long bones and non-traumatic fractures.

Treatment

Cutaneous and most natural food sources of vitamin D are derived from cholecalciferol or vitamin D3. Supplements may be derived from ergocalciferol (vitamin D2) or cholecalciferol (vitamin D3). Therefore, assays used to assess 25-OH-vitamin D levels should measure both D2 and D3, and attention should be paid to the total level of 25-OH-vitamin D, combining the two forms.

Vitamin D3 is two to four times more potent than vitamin D2 on a per unit basis to maintain 25-OH-vitD levels (Misra et al. 2008). However, official guidelines for supplementation do not differentiate between vitamin D2 and D3. It is therefore preferable to treat vitamin D deficient patients with vitamin D3 to more rapidly correct the deficiency. Non-ambulatory children who are vitamin D deficient or insufficient should be treated with 1000–2000IU/day of cholecalciferol (or higher if required). Response to supplementation should be evaluated in 6 months with annual monitoring of serum 25-OH-vitD thereafter.

BONE HEALTH IN NEUROMUSCULAR CONDITIONS

Bones typically grow quickly throughout childhood and adolescence, achieving approximately 90% of adult or peak bone mass, by the third decade of life (Bonjour et al. 1991; Heaney et al. 2000). Peak bone mineral accretion rates occur on average at age 12.5 for girls and 14.0 for boys, resulting in 40–60% of adult bone mass being accrued during the adolescent years. If the attainment of peak bone mass is compromised during childhood or adolescence, there is greater risk for fracture and osteoporosis later in life (Melton et al. 1989; Hui et al. 1990).

Bones adapt based on need, changing internal architecture and shape. In childhood, modelling and remodelling results in increasing bone size and accrual of bone mineral content and density over time. Remodelling is required for repair and maintenance, and through remodelling, calcium and phosphorus are liberated from bone to be used for body functions. This modelling and remodelling occurs continuously throughout life, and is determined by forces on the bone, by genetics and by other modifiable factors. Modifiable determinants of bone mass include overall nutritional intake (particularly of calcium and vitamin D); exercise and lifestyle behaviours; hormonal status; and body weight. Children typically accrue new bone at a greater rate than they lose through remodelling. During adult years, bone mass is usually maintained, and by the fifth decade of life, the rate of remodelling exceeds the rate of deposition resulting in bone loss in later adulthood.

In children with neuromuscular conditions such as cerebral palsy (CP), a combination of atypical muscle tone combined with lack of weight bearing contributes to differences in bone growth and development. Reduced periosteal expansion of lower extremity long bones is a result of the atypical muscle tone and lack of load bearing frequently experienced in children with severe CP. In tibiae of children with CP who are unable to stand or load the bones of their lower extremities, structural differences have been noted: the bones that develop are smaller and thinner (Binkley et al. 2005). Non- and minimally ambulatory children with CP have lower tibial cross-sectional area and cortical bone area than children with CP who can walk (Wren et al. 2011). In addition to the structural differences, the rate of bone accrual is lower in children with severe CP compared to typically developing, weight-bearing children (Henderson et al. 2005). It is important to note that approximately 40% of children with CP were born preterm, and very preterm infants are born at risk for mineral deficiency and metabolic bone disease. This is due to multiple factors, including missing much (or all) of the third trimester in utero when most mineral accretion occurs, inadequate nutrition and mineral intake and frequent illnesses during the neonatal period, lack of movement due to sedation, and exposure to drugs that can negatively impact bone mineralisation such as diuretics and steroids (Bishop & Fewtrell 2003).

People with neurodisabilities may have mild to significant risk for compromised bone health, depending on the degree of medical involvement and nature of their medical condition. Table 8.3 outlines factors that contribute to bone health problems. Fractures in children with severe neuromuscular conditions (such as CP) occur with little or no trauma and most frequently occur in the lower extremities (Mughal 2014). Once a child has sustained a fragility fracture, they are at even higher risk of sustaining additional fractures (Henderson et al. 2002; Goulding et al. 2005; Stevenson et al. 2006).

Assessment of Bone Health

Assessment of bone density allows for quantification of one aspect of bone health, and to identify patients who have compromised bone status and increased risk for fracture. Monitoring bone density allows practitioners the ability to observe change over time, to monitor treatment and to guide clinical decision making.

Several imaging modalities are used to measure bone density and they have advantages and disadvantages. Table 8.4 outlines bone density assessment techniques. For every imaging modality mentioned, patient movement during the image acquisition can negatively impact the quality of the scan and therefore diminish or entirely negate the value of the information yielded by the study. It can be very challenging for children and anyone with a movement disorder to stay still during imaging studies, particularly if the study takes minutes rather than seconds to acquire, if the machine itself is scary looking or sounding, or if the position the patient is required to hold is uncomfortable.

It is important to clarify the definition of density and the way it is used in the field of bone assessment. Density is mass per unit volume of a substance. In the case of bones,

Table 8.3 Contributory factors to compromised bone health

Factor	Mechanism	Effect
Lack of weight bearing	Bones that are unloaded, immobilised, or which have limited to no weight bearing are weaker and less mineralised than load-bearing bones.	In non-ambulatory children, the long bones of the lower extremities are long and thin compared with those of a typically developing weight-bearing child. Bone morphometry is affected by the lack of weight bearing (Binkley et al. 2005; Wren et al. 2011). In adults post spinal cord injury, bones become weaker and more prone to fracture (Abherhalden et al. 2017).
Compromised nutritional status	Poor growth and mineralisation throughout childhood. Specific nutrient deficiencies, especially vitamin D.	Poor BMD and increased risk for fracture.
Medication use (chronic use of anticonvulsants, steroids, antidepressants, proton pump inhibitor and depot medroxyprogesterone acetate)	Can have negative effect on nutrient absorption, metabolism and/or excretion.	Negative effects on BMD have been reported (Leonard et al. 2004; von Scheven et al. 2006; Rahman & Berenson 2010; Ito & Jensen 2012; Beerhorst et al. 2013; Rabenda et al. 2013).
Prior fracture	Fracture with minimal trauma is an indicator of bone quality.	Children who sustain a low-impact fracture are more likely to sustain another fracture (Henderson et al. 2002; Goulding et al. 2005; Stevenson et al. 2006).
Lack of sun exposure/ highly pigmented skin	Vitamin D deficiency.	Undermineralisation of bone.

the density is the amount of mineral in a unit volume. A true density measurement is volumetric or three-dimensional. However, with dual energy X-ray absorptiometry (DXA) instruments, a two-dimensional or areal density is acquired.

DXA is the 'criterion standard' tool for measuring and assessing bone density. Various body sites are recommended for measurement depending on age (Crabtree et al. 2014); body sites to measure by DXA include total body less head, lumbar spine, proximal femur, forearm and the lateral distal femur. In people with neuromuscular conditions, the lateral distal femur (LDF) DXA is often the only body site that can be reliably measured because of the presence of metallic or other non-removable hardware, positioning limitations and involuntary movements (Kecskemethy & Harcke 2014) (Fig. 8.1). In addition, because the lower extremities are at highest risk for fracture in patients who are non-weight bearing, the LDF DXA is the most clinically relevant site to measure.

Table 8.4 Bone densitometry imaging modalities

Modality	Description	Pro	Con
Dual Energy X-ray Absorptiometry (DXA)	DXA uses two different (dual) energy X-ray beams (high- and low-energy photons) to discern soft tissue from bone. DXA is the preferred and most widely available tool used to assess BMD and bone mineral content in adults and children worldwide.	Widely available, low cost, quick, low radiation, high reproducibility. Preferred method to measure BMD worldwide. Normative values across ages are available for all manufacturers and standard protocols are available for all body sites.	Areal measure of bone (2D) measured in gm/cm²; BMD results are affected by bone size (Carter et al. 1992; Prentice et al. 1994; Cole et al. 2005). Scans acquired on machines from different manufacturers are not comparable.
Peripheral Quantitative Computed Tomography (QCT)	Computed tomography machine used to measure the peripheral skeleton, typically of the forearm or tibia. It yields a volumetric measure of BMD in gm/cm³ and provides measures of bone geometry, bone mineral content and estimates of bone strength.	The radiation produced by peripheral QCT is low depending on settings. Yields true volumetric density measurement.	Measurement and assessment protocols vary by institution for the measurement sites, and normative data are limited. Peripheral QCT is not widely available, and its use is generally limited to research applications.
High Resolution Peripheral Quantitative Computed Tomography (HR-pQCT)	CT machine that allows for very high-resolution discernment of internal microstructure and bone macrostructure as well as providing information about BMD and estimates of bone strength.	The greatest amount of detail currently available about bones in vivo is provided by this technology with very low dose exposure to radiation.	Expensive with limited availability; limited to research uses.
Magnetic Resonance Imaging (MRI)	MRI is traditionally used to assess soft tissue, though information about bone can be obtained.	It is a non-radiation imaging modality that yields volumetric measures. Like QCT, MRI provides information on volumetric bone density and bone geometry.	Use is limited as an evaluative technique for bone densitometry. Protocols are not well developed for use in children or adults with neuromuscular disabilities, normative bone density data are not available, and because the instruments are so frequently used for other indications, it can be difficult to get time on the scanner. Use is currently limited to research.

(continued on next page)

Table 8.4 Bone densitometry imaging modalities (continued)

Modality	Description	Pro	Con
Quantitative Ultrasound (QUS)	Attenuation and velocity of sound waves are measured by ultrasound. Speed of sound and attenuation are affected by the distribution of cortical bone, and because there are changes in the two types of bone during growth, interpreting QUS measures can be especially challenging in children.	Machines are affordable and portable, and ultrasound does not produce any radiation. Limited normative data are available. Several different devices are available that measure differing body sites and utilise different ultrasound techniques.	Qualitative ultrasound does not give a bone density measurement and is not a proxy for other methods of measuring bone density (Christoforidis et al. 2011; Williams et al. 2012). QUS is used as a screening tool in the USA.

Published normative values are available for the LDF DXA, though they are currently limited to one manufacturer's machine (Zemel et al. 2009).

Familiarity with both DXA measurement techniques and the population being measured will dictate the quality and success of the scan. Table 8.5 outlines common conditions encountered when measuring children with disabilities by DXA and the effect on the DXA.

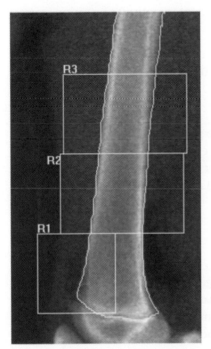

Figure 8.1 The lateral distal femur DXA analysis provides information on three regions of interest: R1 is primarily trabecular bone (metaphyseal); R2 is a mixture of trabecular and cortical bone (metadiaphyseal); and R3 is primarily cortical (diaphyseal).

Table 8.5 Common medical issues encountered in children with disabilities, effect on DXA, and DXA site affected (Reprint with permission Kecskemethy & Harcke 2014)

Medical condition	Problem created with scan	DXA site affected
Excessive movement	Movement artefact	All; least likely to affect LDF
Contractures	Inability to place correct regions of interest	TB; H
Scoliosis	Inability to place correct regions of interest	TB; LS
Metallic implant	Artefact – metal adds density	All; implants least likely in LDF
Feeding tube	Artefact – adds density or area	
Baclofen pump	Artefact – metal adds density	TB; likely LS
High muscle tone	Positioning problems; unable to lie flat	TB; possibly LS
Startle reflex	Movement artefact when table and/or arm moves	TB; H; rarely LDF
Obesity	Patient exceeds width of table	All; most likely TB
Cognitive delays	Patient unable to understand instructions	TB
Dislocated hip	Atypical anatomy invalidates landmarks for valid analysis	All; most likely TB H; possibly LDF

TB = total body; LS = lumbar spine; H = hip; LDF = lateral distal femur

Consideration of the conditions commonly encountered when measuring DXA in patients with disabilities will help to guide the imaging centre on scan acquisition and interpretation. It is very important to keep in mind that for accurate and valid testing of bone density in neurodisabling conditions, specially trained imaging specialists should be consulted. If such expertise is not available, it is prudent to optimise nutrition, correct deficiencies and treat based on clinical findings.

Prevention and Treatment for Compromised Bone Health

NUTRITION

Addressing nutrition should be part of a preventive programme for any child or adult with physical disabilities. Assuring adequate intake of minerals and vitamins, either by diet alone, or with supplements, should be part of the routine evaluation by care providers. In addition, serum vitamin D levels need to be assessed yearly, with a target level of 30–50ng/mL for 25-OH-vitamin D.

WEIGHT BEARING

Everyone with neurodisabilities should be encouraged to weight bear and ambulate as much as possible to strengthen bone. Those with disabilities who are able to ambulate (whether unaided or with the help of braces, crutches or a walker) should be encouraged to do so as tolerated. While there is no evidence as to how much weight bearing is 'enough' to protect against the development of osteoporosis, doing so as much and as often as possible, with regularity, seems prudent.

VIBRATION

There are two main ways of providing vibration therapy: whole body vibration and low intensity vibration or low magnitude mechanical stimulation. These two types of vibration differ and while both have been studied in animals and humans, the impact on BMD in children with neurodisabilities is inconsistent (Rubin et al. 2004; Wren et al. 2010; Ruck et al. 2010).

MEDICATIONS

If appropriate nutrition and weight bearing have been achieved and the patient develops a fragility fracture in the face of low bone density, that patient should be treated with medication. In adults, it is standard practice to initiate treatment for low BMD based on bone density results alone; however, there is no consensus for this practice in children. Some practitioners initiate pharmacological treatment based on low BMD alone in children who are at high risk for fracture, while others initiate treatment after the occurrence of a fragility fracture.

When treatment with medications is indicated, this usually means bisphosphonates (BPs) in children, whereas in adults, it can mean a number of possibilities, including BPs.

Bisphosphonates

BPs act by inhibiting osteoclast function, thus slowing bone resorption. They have been used to treat osteoporosis for many years, with good evidence for safety and efficacy. While many of these studies have been in adults, there is good evidence for their effectiveness in treating children with osteogenesis imperfecta, CP and muscular dystrophy (Bachrach et al. 2010; Sbrocchi et al. 2012; Feehan et al. 2018). In children, intravenous formulations of BPs are typically used (pamidronate or zoledronic acid), whereas in adults, the oral forms are frequently used (alendronate, risedronate or ibandronate). BP treatment should only begin with a sufficient vitamin D level and a normal serum calcium and phosphorus, as hypocalcaemia and hypophosphataemia are among the more common side effects. Optimal length of treatment for children is not known, but in children with neurodisabilities is usually a minimum of 1–2 years. In adults, length of treatment is up to 5 years, followed by a drug holiday due to concerns of the development of atypical femur fractures. A potential serious side effect is development of osteonecrosis of the jaw, to date only reported in adults.

Denosumab

A RANK-L inhibitor, denosumab blocks the development of osteoclasts. It is approved for use in post-menopausal women at risk for osteoporosis both by the Food and Drug Administration (FDA) in the USA and by the Committee for Medicinal Products for Human Use (CHMP) in Europe. It is given monthly or every 6 months by subcutaneous injection. Increasingly, denosumab is used in adults with CP and other neurodevelopmental disabilities.

Teriparatide

Teriparatide is a recombinant protein form of PTH. It is an effective anabolic agent, stimulating osteoblastic activity. It has been approved by the US FDA and by the CHMP for use in men and post-menopausal women with osteoporosis at risk for fractures. It is not approved for children or young adults with open epiphyses.

SUMMARY POINTS

1. People with neurodisabilities have mild to significant risk for compromised bone health, depending on the degree of medical involvement and nature of their medical condition.

    a. In children with neuromuscular disease such as CP, a combination of atypical muscle tone combined with lack of weight bearing contributes to differences in bone growth and development, resulting in reduced bone size and bone density.

2. Nutrition:

    a. Nutritional status is directly related to bone health in patients with neuromuscular conditions.

    b. The three most important nutrients for bone health are calcium, phosphorus and vitamin D.

    c. Calcium is not made in the body – it must be ingested and absorbed. Vitamin D ensures effective absorption of dietary calcium.

    d. Nutritional rickets can come about because of sunlight deficiency, dietary deficiency of calcium or vitamin D, malabsorption of calcium, phosphorus or vitamin D, or renal losses of phosphorus and calcium.

3. Vitamin D:

    a. Serum 25-OH-vitamin D results are classified into levels: deficient, insufficient, sufficient and high. Currently, there are two differing recommendations for the classification of serum 25 vitamin D levels.

   b. Even by the stricter criteria, vitamin D deficiency in the general population is quite common, as evidenced by studies from around the world.

4. Two forms of vitamin D are found in supplements: D2 and D3. Vitamin D3 more rapidly corrects deficiency, and is therefore the preferred form to use. Non-ambulatory children who are vitamin D deficient or insufficient should be treated with 1000–2000IU/day of cholecalciferol (or higher if required); response to supplementation should be evaluated in 6 months with annual monitoring of serum 25-OH-vitamin D thereafter.

5. Bone density assessment:

   a. DXA is the 'criterion standard' tool for measuring and assessing bone density.

   b. Various body sites are recommended for measurement depending on age.

   c. The LDF DXA is the most feasible and clinically relevant site to measure in patients with neurodisabilities.

   d. DXA should be performed at an imaging centre familiar with techniques used in measuring patients with neurodisabilities. If such expertise is not available, it is prudent to optimise nutrition, correct deficiencies and treat based on clinical findings

6. Prevention:

   a. Addressing nutrition should be part of a preventive programme for any child or adult with physical disabilities. Assuring adequate intake of minerals and vitamins, either by diet alone, or with supplements, should be part of the routine evaluation by care providers.

   b. Serum vitamin D levels need to be assessed yearly, with a target level of 30–50ng mL for 25-OH-vitamin D.

   c. Weight bearing and ambulation should be encouraged to strengthen bone.

7. Treatment:

   a. In adults, it is standard practice to initiate treatment for low BMD based on bone density results alone.

   b. In children, some physicians treat for low bone density alone, while others treat only after a fragility fracture has occurred.

   c. When treatment with medications is indicated, this usually means BPs in children, whereas in adults it can mean a number of possibilities, including BPs.

REFERENCES

Abderhalden L, Weaver FM, Bethel M et al. (2017) Dual-energy X-ray absorptiometry and fracture prediction in patients with spinal cord injuries and disorders. *Osteoporos Int* 28(3): 925–934. doi: 10.1007/s00198-016-3841-y. Epub 2016 Dec 6.

Bachrach SJ, Kecskemethy HH, Harcke HT, Hossain J (2010) Decreased fracture incidence after one year of pamidronate treatment in children with spastic quadriplegic cerebral palsy. *Dev Med Child Neurol* 52: 837–842.

Beerhorst K, van der Kruijs SJ, Verschuure P, Tan IY, Aldenkamp AP (2013) Bone disease during chronic antiepileptic drug therapy: general versus specific risk factors. *J Neurol Sci* 331(1–2): 19–25. doi: 10.1016/j.jns.2013.05.005.

Beto JA (2015) The role of calcium in human aging. *Clin Nutr Res* 4(1): 1–8. doi: 10.7762/cnr.2015.4.1.1. Epub 2015 Jan 16.

Binkley T, Johnson J, Vogel L, Kecskemethy H, Henderson R, Specker B (2005) Bone measurements by peripheral quantitative computed tomography (pQCT) in children with cerebral palsy. *J Pediatr* 147: 791–796.

Bishop N, Fewtrell M (2003) Metabolic bone disease of prematurity. In: Glorieux FH, Pettifor JM, Juppner H (eds). *Pediatric Bone: Biology and Diseases*. New York: Academic Press, pp 567–581.

Bonjour JP, Theintz G, Buchs B, Slosman D, Rizzoli R (1991) Critical years and stages of puberty for spinal and femoral bone mass accumulation during adolescence. *J Clin Endocrinol Metab* 73: 555–563.

Carter DR, Bouxsein ML, Marcus R (1992) New approaches for interpreting projected bone densitometry data. *J Bone Miner Res* 7(2): 137–145.

Christoforidis A, Printza N, Gkogka C et al. (2011) Comparative study of quantitative ultrasonography and dual-energy X-ray absorptiometry for evaluating renal osteodystrophy in children with chronic kidney disease. *J Bone Miner Metab* 29(3): 321–327. doi: 10.1007/s00774-010-0220-1.

Cole JH, Scerpella TA, van der Meulen MC (2005) Fan-beam densitometry of the growing skeleton: are we measuring what we think we are? *J Clin Densitom* 8(1): 57–64.

Crabtree NJ, Arabi A, Bachrach LK et al. (2014) Dual-energy X-ray absorptiometry interpretation and reporting in children and adolescents: the revised 2013 ISCD official pediatric positions. *J Clin Densitom* 17: 225–242.

Feehan AG, Zacharin MR, Lim AS, Simm PJ (2018) A comparative study of quality of life, functional and bone outcomes in osteogenesis imperfecta with bisphosphonate therapy initiated in childhood or adulthood. *Bone* 113: 137–143. doi: 10.1016/j.bone.2018.05.021. Epub 2018 May 19.

Goulding A, Jones IE, Williams SM et al. (2005) First fracture is associated with increased risk of new fractures during growth. *J Pediatr* 146(2): 286–288.

Händel MN, Heitmann BL, Abrahamsen B (2015) Nutrient and food intakes in early life and risk of childhood fractures: a systematic review and meta-analysis. *Am J Clin Nutr* 102(5): 1182–1195. doi: 10.3945/ajcn.115.108456. Epub 2015 Oct 7.

Heaney RP, Abrams S, Dawson-Hughes B et al. (2000) Peak bone mass. *Osteoporos Int* 11: 985–1009.

Henderson RC, Lark RK, Gurka MJ et al. (2002) Bone density and metabolism in children and adolescents with moderate to severe cerebral palsy. *Pediatrics* 110(1Pt1): e5.

Henderson RC, Kairalla J, Abbas A, Stevenson RD (2004) Predicting low bone density in children and young adults with quadriplegic cerebral palsy. *Dev Med Child Neurol* 46(6): 416–419.

Henderson RC, Gilbert SR, Clement ME, Abbas A, Worley G, Stevenson RD (2005) Altered skeletal maturation in moderate to severe cerebral palsy. *Dev Med Child Neurol* 47(4): 229–236.

Hoge A, Donneau AF, Streel S et al. (2015) Vitamin D deficiency is common among adults in Wallonia (Belgium, 51°30′ North): findings from the Nutrition, Environment and Cardio-Vascular Health study. *Nutr Res* 35(8): 716–725. doi: 10.1016/j.nutres.2015.06.005. Epub 2015 Jun 15.

Holick MF (2004) Sunlight and vitamin D for bone health and prevention of autoimmune diseases, cancers and cardiovascular disease. *Am J Clin Nutr* 80(Suppl 6): 1678S–1688S.

Holick MF, Binkley NC, Bischoff-Ferrari HA et al. (2011) Evaluation, treatment, and prevention of vitamin D deficiency: an Endocrine Society clinical practice guideline. *J Clin Endocrinol Metab* 96(7): 1911–1930. doi: 10.1210/jc.2011-0385. Erratum in: *J Clin Endocrinol Metab* 2011 96(12): 3908.

Hui SL, Slemenda CW, Johnston CC Jr (1990) The contribution of bone loss to postmenopausal osteoporosis. *Osteoporos Int* 1: 30–34.

Institute of Medicine, Food and Nutrition Board (2010) *Dietary Reference Intakes for Calcium and Vitamin D*. Washington, DC: National Academy Press.

Ito T, Jensen RT (2010) Association of long-term proton pump inhibitor therapy with bone fractures and effects on absorption of calcium, vitamin B12, iron, and magnesium. *Curr Gastroenterol Rep* 12(6): 448–457. doi: 10.1007/s11894-010-0141-0.

Kecskemethy HH, Harcke HT (2014) Assessment of bone health in children with disabilities. *J Pediatr Rehabil Med* 7(2): 111–124. doi: 10.3233/PRM-140280.

Leonard MB, Feldman HI, Shults J, Zemel BS, Foster BJ, Stallings VA (2004) Long-term, high-dose glucocorticoids and bone mineral content in childhood glucocorticoid-sensitive nephrotic syndrome. *N Engl J Med* 351(9): 868–875.

Liu X, Baylin A, Levy PD (2018) Vitamin D deficiency and insufficiency among US adults: prevalence, predictors and clinical implications. *Br J Nutr* 119(8): 928–936. doi: 10.1017/S0007114518000491.

Manios Y, Moschonis G, Hulshof T et al. (2017) Prevalence of vitamin D deficiency and insufficiency among schoolchildren in Greece: the role of sex, degree of urbanization and seasonality. *Br J Nutr* 118(7): 550–558. doi: 10.1017/S0007114517002422. Epub 2017 Oct 2.

Mazidi M, Kengne AP, Vatanparast H (2018) Association of dietary patterns of American adults with bone mineral density and fracture. *Public Health Nutr* 21(13): 2417–2423. doi: 10.1017/S1368980018000939. Epub 2018 May 21.

Misra M, Pacaud D, Petryk A et al. (2008) Vitamin D deficiency in children and its management: review of current knowledge and recommendations. *Pediatrics* 122: 398–417.

Melton LJ, Kan SH, Frye MA, Wahner HW, O'Fallon WM, Riggs BL (1989) Epidemiology of vertebral fractures in women. *Am J Epidemiol* 129: 1000–1111.

Mughal MZ (2014) Fractures in children with CP. *Current Osteoporo Rep* 12: 313–318.

Prentice A, Parsons TJ, Cole TJ (1994) Uncritical use of bone mineral density in absorptiometry may lead to size-related artifacts in the identification of bone mineral determinants. *Am J Clin Nutr* 60(6): 837–842.

Priemel M, von Domarus C, Klatte TO et al. (2010) Bone mineralization defects and vitamin D deficiency: histomorphometric analysis of iliac crest bone biopsies and circulating 25-hydroxyvitamin D in 675 patients. *J Bone Miner Res* 25: 305–312.

Rabenda V, Nicolet D, Beaudart C, Bruyère O, Reginster JY (2013) Relationship between use of antidepressants and risk of fractures: a meta-analysis. *Osteoporos Int* 24(1): 121–137.

Rahman M, Berenson AB (2010) Predictors of higher bone mineral density loss and use of depot medroxyprogesterone acetate. *Obstet Gynecol* 115(1): 35–40. doi: 0.1097/AOG.0b013e3181c4e864.

Rubin C, Recker R, Cullen D, Ryaby J, McCabe J, Mcleod K (2004) Prevention of postmenopausal bone loss by a low-magnitude, high-frequency mechanical stimuli: a clinical trial assessing compliance, efficacy, and safety. *J Bone Miner Res* 19: 343–351.

Ruck J, Chabot G, Rauch F (2010) Vibration treatment in cerebral palsy: a randomized controlled pilot study. *J Musculoskelet Neuronal Interact* 10(1): 77–83.

Sbrocchi AM, Rauch F, Jacob P et al. (2012) The use of intravenous bisphosphonate therapy to treat vertebral fractures due to osteoporosis among boys with Duchenne muscular dystrophy. *Osteoporos Int* 23(11): 2703–2711.

Stevenson RD, Conaway M, Barrington JW, Cuthill SL, Worley G, Henderson RC (2006) Fracture rate in children with cerebral palsy. *Pediatric Rehabil* 9(4): 396–403.

von Scheven E, Gordon CM, Wypij D, Wertz M, Gallagher KT, Bachrach L (2006) Variable deficits of bone mineral despite chronic glucocorticoid therapy in pediatric patients with inflammatory diseases: a Glaser Pediatric Research Network study. *J Pediatr Endocrinol Metab* 19(6): 821–830.

Webb AR, Kazantzidis A, Kift RC et al. (2018a) Colour counts: sunlight and skin type as drivers of vitamin D deficiency at UK latitudes. *Nutrients* 10(4): 457. doi: 10.3390/nu10040457.

Webb AR, Kazantzidis A, Kift RC et al. (2018b) Meeting vitamin D requirements in white Caucasians at UK latitudes: providing a choice. *Nutrients* 10(4): pii: E497. doi: 10.3390/nu10040497.

Williams JE, Wilson CM, Biassoni L, Suri R, Fewtrell MS (2012) Dual energy x-ray absorptiometry and quantitative ultrasound are not interchangeable in diagnosing abnormal bones. *Arch Dis Child* 97(9): 822–824. doi: 10.1136/archdischild-2011-301326.

Wren TA, Lee DC, Hara R et al. (2010) Effect of high-frequency, low-magnitude vibration on bone and muscle in children with cerebral palsy. *J Pediatr Orthop* 30(7): 732–738.

Wren TA, Lee DC, Kay RM, Dorey FJ, Gilsanz V (2011) Bone density and size in ambulatory children with cerebral palsy. *Dev Med Child Neurol* 53(2): 137–141.

Zemel BS, Stallings VA, Leonard MB et al. (2009) Revised pediatric reference data for the lateral distal femur measured by Hologic Discovery/Delphi dual energy x-ray absorptiometry. *J Clin Densitom* 12: 207–218.

CHAPTER 9

Feeding and Nutritional Management Strategies

Kristie L Bell, Katherine A Benfer and Kelly A Weir

INTRODUCTION

Comprehensive nutritional assessment and management is complex for children with neurological impairment (NI). Poor nutritional status is common and may arise from a variety of causes (Ptomey & Wittenbrook 2015). Many children have oropharyngeal dysphagia (feeding and swallowing difficulties) with subsequent increased risk of pulmonary aspiration and poor respiratory health. Prolonged and stressful feeding results in difficulty consuming adequate food and fluids to maintain good nutritional status, hydration and overall health (Arvedson 2013). As detailed in Chapter 4, gastrointestinal disorders including foregut dysmotility, gastroesophageal reflux disease, delayed gastric emptying and constipation are frequent and can have significant impacts on dietary intakes. Energy requirements are variable; they can be increased for children with high levels of involuntary movements and decreased for those with spasticity and reduced mobility (see Chapter 7). For some children with NI, there is a significant behavioural component to feeding resulting in poor energy intake or imbalanced micronutrient intake and subsequent micronutrient deficiencies.

THE MULTIDISCIPLINARY TEAM IN THE NUTRITIONAL MANAGEMENT OF A CHILD WITH NEURODISABILITY

Given the complex aetiology of poor nutrition for children with NI, assessment of nutritional status should be conducted by a multidisciplinary team (MDT) with a range of knowledge, skills and expertise; assessment should also use multiple methodologies (Ptomey & Wittenbrook, 2015; Romano et al. 2017). Thorough, coordinated evaluation and treatment planning are essential for successful interventions.

The MDT brings together professionals from multiple disciplines to address the child's nutritional status and requirements, feeding and swallowing function, gastrointestinal function, and the child and family's social and emotional needs. This includes the prescription and administration of interventions as well as ongoing monitoring and adjustment of treatments as required.

MDT membership may be highly variable depending on location and available resources, and may include paediatricians, dietitians, speech pathologists, gastroenterologists, surgeons, radiologists, nurses, social workers, psychologists, occupational therapists, physiotherapists, educators, respite carers, and social and community supports. Central to the team are the child's family and primary caregivers whose involvement ensures that interventions are individualised, realistic, targeted, take into account the child's individual preferences, socio-cultural aspects, family and environment factors, and will have the greatest likelihood of success (Craig et al. 2003).

NUTRITIONAL INTERVENTIONS

Given the high prevalence of oropharyngeal dysphagia and undernutrition, interventions for children with NI are frequently focused on increasing nutritional intake to improve nutritional status and overall health (Bell & Samson-Fang 2013; Romano et al. 2017). Interventions can range from relatively straightforward correction of micronutrient deficiencies in children who are able to consume a full range of food and fluid textures without difficulty, to complete enteral tube feeding in those unable to protect their airway during swallowing across all food and fluid textures. **Oral nutrition support** includes strategies to support the child's mealtime environment and positioning, alterations to food/fluid textures and nutrient density, and use of adaptive equipment, caregiver techniques and sensorimotor therapy. **Enteral tube feeding** can be the sole source of nutrition or can be used as an adjunct to oral nutrition support. A simplified decision making tree for determining oral feeding versus tube feeding is shown in Figure 9.1.

This decision tree can be considered in conjunction with a management hierarchy that emphasises the importance and interplay between outcomes of safety, efficiency, skill development and mealtime stress, considered in the sociocultural context (Fig. 9.2).

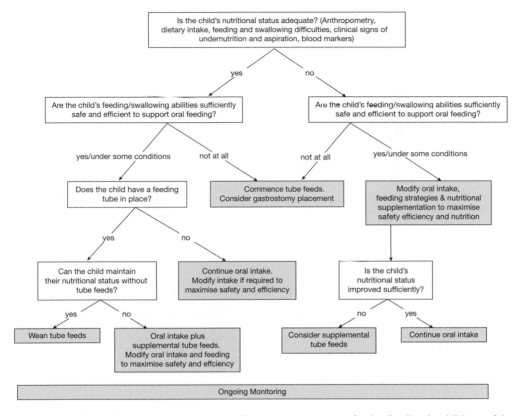

Figure 9.1 Simplified decision-making tree for commencement of tube feeding in children with neurological impairment.

Oral Nutrition Support

Initial intervention for a child who is able to achieve functional feeding and swallowing skills and airway protection will involve a trial of oral nutrition support strategies. Approaches to support oral intake include alterations to food and fluid textures and nutrient density as well as strategies to support the child's mealtime environment, feeding position, adaptive equipment, caregiver techniques and oral sensorimotor therapy. These approaches are commonly combined to holistically support the child's mealtime safety, efficiency and success; but specific aspects may differ depending on the target outcome.

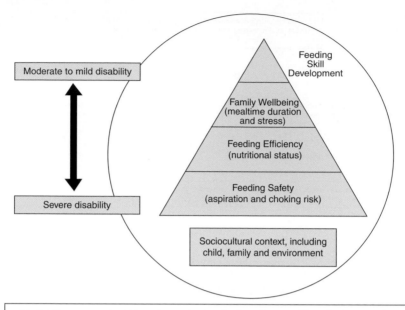

The feeding management hierarchy emphasises the importance and interplay between the outcomes (goals and management prioritiers) of feeding safety and efficiency, mealtime stress and feeding skill development, all in a sociocultural context. Feeding safety is the base of the pyramid and initial consideration, with progression upwards to reflect the order of priorities for oral feeding up to skill development at the top. Feeding Skill Development includes developmental progression of ingestion skills, food and/or fluid textures and utensils.

Figure 9.2 Feeding management hierarchy.

OPTIMISING THE MEALTIME ENVIRONMENT AND ROUTINES

Mealtimes form a central and significant part of family life, and attempts should be made to ensure positive experiences for both the child and the caregiver (Morris & Klein 2000). The primary foundations for mealtime success are to ensure the child's readiness to feed, and to provide a safe, predictable and responsive environment. Depending on the child's pre-mealtime physiological state, either a calming or alerting environment can be facilitated for the child by altering aspects such as temperature, light, visual stimuli (including colour and contrast of utensils) and auditory inputs (Morris & Klein 2000). Minimising environmental distractions should balance maintaining the child's attention whilst encouraging the social aspects of a mealtime.

More complex food/fluid textures should be included in mealtimes when the child is most alert, interested and feeds most effectively. Children with moderate oral motor involvement may benefit from smaller more frequent meals during the day, limited to 30–40 minutes duration (Reau et al. 1996). Mealtime schedules may need to be flexible and responsive to the day-to-day variability in the child's mealtime performance, and also energy fluctuations and fatigue through the day.

A predictable mealtime routine can help children with mealtime expectations (including cultural behaviours such as sitting at the table), particularly for children with cognitive/learning difficulties, impaired vision or hearing. Children can better prepare their body and cognition for the approaching meal if provided with consistent mealtime signals, such as presenting their spoon visually/tactilely, or with consistent verbal cues. Other aspects include a consistent feeder (particularly in institutional settings), consistent positioning and consistent utensils (Burklow et al. 2002). Consistent verbal and visual cues can remind children of specific ingestion functions or behaviours, such as 'single bites' or 'chew and swallow'.

Developing the child's ability to effectively communicate (through formal or informal communication systems), and the caregiver's sensitivity and responsiveness to the child's cues, assists the child to express food preferences, enjoyment, pain or discomfort, and their desire to continue or cease the meal (Mathisen et al. 1989). A focus on the child–caregiver interactions during mealtimes also facilitates the rich language and social learning opportunities a mealtime avails.

Postural Management and Positioning when Eating

Optimal positioning to improve head and trunk stability during mealtimes provides a critical foundation for both safety and efficiency, and is a priority for all children with feeding difficulties (Benfer et al. 2013). Optimal mealtime positioning influences tone and overall patterns of movement, improves coordination of oral motor movements, enhances respiration and airway protection, provides a mechanical advantage for bolus dynamics, positively influences reflux and gut motility, and improves self-feeding (Hulme et al. 1983). Modification of a child's sitting position from one of generalised extension to greater flexion (particularly at the hips and knees) can facilitate jaw stability and head flexion (Stratten 1981). A stable and aligned head position, achieved both through overall body positioning and specific head support (including head rests or occipital rolls), may improve position, mobility and coordination of the lips, tongue and oral anatomy (Lanert & Ekberg 1995).

Ideal mealtime positioning involves the child seated upright, with 90-degree hip flexion, feet supported, head in midline and aligned on the anterior–posterior plane, and chin slightly tucked. However, no single optimal position exists for all children. Recommendations for mealtime position should be made in collaboration with the child's physical or occupational therapist, incorporating individualised findings from videofluoroscopy when appropriate and available (Lanert & Ekberg 1995; Gisel et al. 2003). Options for improving mealtime positioning may include specialised seating (infant feeder seats, wheelchairs or supportive chairs); the adaptation of regular seating using pillows, rolled towels, foam and support straps; or postural support by the caregiver's body. A tray may provide additional postural support and allow stabilisation of the upper limb and shoulder girdle, to achieve a functional sitting position (Stavness 2006). Whilst an upright position is generally advocated, up to 30 degrees of recline, for children who are unstable in an upright position, reduces lip pursing, gag and tongue thrust (Lanert & Ekberg 1995). The upright position may be more beneficial than recline for children with poor pharyngeal clearance or those requiring a slower bolus flow rate (Morton et al. 1993). Flexed head position and chin tuck improves protection of the airway, decreases risk of laryngeal penetration and aspiration and is particularly helpful for children with a delayed swallow initiation (Lanert & Ekberg 1995). Preliminary evidence suggests that reductions in aspiration from improved position, combined with texture modification of food and fluids, translate into longer-term improvements in respiratory function for children with severe feeding difficulties (Gisel et al. 2003).

CAREGIVER MEALTIME TECHNIQUES

Training parents in techniques including provision of jaw and cheek support, appropriate bolus size and placement in the mouth, and pacing techniques can be highly effective for improving the child's mealtime safety and efficiency. In addition, the consistent incorporation of behavioural strategies by caregivers, into all meals and snacks, provides maximum opportunities to enhance mealtime success. Behavioural training approaches aim to reduce feeding behaviours related to food refusal and selective eating (Sharp et al. 2010). While strong evidence exists for their use in certain subgroups of children, it is critical when using behavioural strategies with children with NI that underlying oral sensorimotor and gastrointestinal issues are resolved in parallel (Morris & Klein 2000). Behavioural strategies can be understood broadly as (1) operant training approaches, which aim to increase or decrease specific mealtime behaviours through positive and negative reinforcement (Babbitt et al. 1994); (2) behavioural approaches to skill acquisition, which simplify the mealtime task to aid learning, and may include shaping, prompting and modelling (Babbitt et al. 1994); and (3) food chaining and systematic desensitisation hierarchies which aim to gradually expose the child to new mealtime experiences, particularly tastes, textures or foods by building on the child's existing food repertoire in a gradual stepwise method (Toomey & Ross 2011).

Provision of jaw and/or cheek support can effectively create a base of stability for the lips, tongue and cheeks, thereby enhancing mealtime efficiency. There are many detailed accounts on types of oral support in dedicated mealtime texts (Morris & Klein 2000; Winstock 2005) which have demonstrated effectiveness in infants and young children (Hwang et al. 2010). Jaw support may not be necessary if the child can be adequately positioned in a neutral-flexed posture, and so should be considered secondary to optimal seated positioning. While maladaptive oral patterns may be reduced through provision of jaw/cheek support, careful consideration must be given to the function of the oral pattern for ingestion (e.g. forward–back tongue pattern may be necessary for oral transport).

Bolus size may be manipulated by the caregiver specific to the properties associated with the bolus consistency (e.g. fluid or chewable), and depending on the particular oral sensorimotor difficulties of the child (Arvedson 1998). Large boluses have been associated with an increased risk of aspiration in children with NI, and so limiting spoon and bite size is recommended (Mirrett et al. 1994). However, bolus size should be individually evaluated in the context of the child's oral sensorimotor skills, because larger bolus volumes may provide greater sensory input to the mouth (allowing for improved bolus formation and transit) (Arvedson 1998), and decrease pharyngeal delay times in adults with dysphagia (Bisch et al. 1994).

Specific bolus placement techniques differ depending on the texture of the bolus, utensil used, and the child's individual oral sensorimotor skills and goals. Generally, for foods given via spoon, presentation from the midline and chest level upward will promote alignment of the head and a chin tuck position. Touching the spoon to the child's lips can alert them to the oncoming bolus and encourage mouth opening. Gentle downward pressure can be provided through the spoon to the tongue to provide sensory feedback and may inhibit tongue thrust (Helfrich-Miller et al. 1986). The caregiver can be encouraged to allow adequate time for upper lip clearance of the spoon, and to gently tilt the spoon to make contact with the upper lip (Helfrich-Miller et al. 1986). Chewable or lumpy foods may be more appropriately placed laterally, over the molars to encourage mastication. This is particularly important for children with reduced tongue lateralisation to ensure food is adequately chewed for the swallow, thereby reducing any risk of choking.

Slowing the pace of the meal by incorporating pauses between boluses allows the child time to breathe and re-establish their feeding rhythm (Arvedson 1998) and ensures adequate time to clear the bolus (from the oral cavity and pharynx) before subsequent boluses are presented (Logemann 1998). Specific strategies can include teaching caregivers to count the number of sucks when bottle feeding before tilting the bottle for a breath, and helping the caregiver learn to observe the timing of the swallow (through visual or tactile means) (Law-Morstatt et al. 2003). Using information gained from instrumental assessments can provide caregivers with specific strategies to aid their child.

Adaptive Equipment

Utensils: Depending on the child's developmental age and oropharyngeal swallowing skill, a range of feeding utensils may be used to provide nutrition safely and efficiently, and to assist in the development of feeding and swallowing skills. If a child is breastfed, the mother can use equipment such as nipple shields and supplementary feeders to enhance feeding outcomes. A range of nipples/teats, spoons, forks, knives and cups are available which can be matched to the child's specific oropharyngeal swallow function. A short discussion of these is presented in Table 9.1 (Morris & Klein 2000).

Table 9.1 Features of feeding utensils

Utensil	Feature	Explanation
Nipples/ Teats	Number of holes	Holes usually drip at a given rate for a specific age group (e.g. Premmie teat for below term age; slow flow: 0–3 months; medium flow: 4–6 months; fast flow: over 6 months of age). However, flow rates can be highly variable across brands, due to type of material and bottle construction.
	Slit or Y cut	Non-drip teats which open to allow fluid flow when child is actively sucking and close during suck-pauses. These are helpful for children with reduced respiratory support/stamina.
	Variable flow	Provides a range of flow rates depending upon the orientation of the teat with the child's nose.
		Allows for feeder to change flow rates during the feed to respond to child's suck swallow breathe coordination and stamina/fatigue.
Bottles	Squeeze bottles	Soft silicon or 'squeeze' bottles allow feeder to provide pressure to the bottle to support fluid flow for a child with a weak suck. Feeder must coordinate squeeze with child's sucking and stop during suck-pauses or rests.
	Sports bottles	Often popular as non-spill bottles; however, they present an aspiration risk as children often drink from sports bottles with their head tilted back and their neck extended. This posture opens their airway and results in frequent coughing during drinking. Bottles with straws allow the child to maintain chin tuck or a neutral head position for better airway safety.
Cups	Straw cups	Encourages chin tuck position which supports more active airway protection. Requires good lip closure, cheek strength and palate closure to create and sustain negative oral pressure and suction.
	Spout cups	If spout cup without a valve is used, this allows flow of fluid for child with poor oral suction and controls the volume/flow rate. If a valve is used, the child must be able to create negative suction pressure to extract fluid.
		Penetration-aspiration risk if head is tipped back to get fluid from bottom of the cup.
	Open cup	Developmental target. Child must be able to maintain a stable jaw position and bottom lip contact with the cup. Curved surface on the cup rim will enhance lip–rim contact. This cup is good for thickened fluids.
	Cut-out cup	Rim of cup is cut out on the top surface. Allows the child to drink from the cup whilst maintaining a chin tuck or neutral head position by allowing cup tilt with space for the nose.
Spoons	Shallow bowl	Requires less active upper lip closure to remove bolus from spoon. Helpful for children with lip weakness.
	Deep bowl	Requires more active lip closure/pressure and may provide a bigger bolus.
	Broad base	Enables feeder to use deep pressure sensory input with spoon presentation to minimise tongue protrusion and encourage containment of the tongue within the oral cavity.
Forks/ Knives	Built up handles	Forks, knives and spoons with curved or built up handles may be suitable for young children or those with upper limb motor involvement and grip difficulties. These may aid independent eating and development of utensil use.

OTHER THERAPEUTIC TECHNIQUES

Oral Sensorimotor Treatment (OSMT) is commonly used in children with NI and dysphagia as part of a comprehensive management programme, although efficacy research has focused on moderate–severely physically impaired children. OSMT includes specific tasks using food to improve oral musculature strength, precision and range of movement to support the functional aspects of the oral phase of swallowing. Improvements such as lip closure during spoon feeding, straw drinking and chewing, tongue lateralisation during chewing, bolus containment, shorter chewing time and faster oral transfer have been demonstrated. No improvement to suction strength during straw drinking, the pharyngeal phase of swallowing (e.g. aspiration or post-swallow pharyngeal residue), mealtime efficiency or weight gain have been shown (Gisel 1996; Snider et al. 2011; Kaviyani Baghbadorani et al. 2014). Functional Chewing Training (Inal et al. 2017) has had promising results in improving chewing function by positioning food or a chewing tube to the molar area to stimulate lateral and rotary tongue movements, massage the upper and lower gums, and gradually increase food consistency. Specific oral sensorimotor treatment strategies and activities for various types of oral motor dysfunction during feeding are described extensively elsewhere (Morris & Klein 2000).

ROBOTIC ASSISTIVE FEEDING DEVICES, ORAL APPLIANCES AND USE OF NEUROMUSCULAR ELECTRICAL STIMULATION

Robotic assistive feeding devices such as the 'Robotic Aid to Eating' support independent feeding and consistent food presentation via a spoon to enhance feeding skills and efficiency. Improvements in mastication and swallowing have been found whilst using the device, but not retained over time. No benefits for energy or protein consumption, increased food intake, weight gain or feeding efficiency have been noted (Snider et al. 2011). Use of an intraoral appliance such as the Innsbruck Sensorimotor Activator and Regulator (ISMAR) includes the fitting of an intraoral appliance specifically fabricated on the child's own dental cast. Moderate evidence supports use of the ISMAR to improve oral postural control and oral sensorimotor skills such as spoon feeding, biting and chewing, and cup and straw drinking compared to no or alternate therapies, but there is less evidence to show positive effects in time taken for meals (feeding efficiency) or weight gain (Snider et al. 2011). Neuromuscular Electrical Stimulation (NMES) treatment is an emerging treatment option involving neuromuscular electrical stimulation via bipolar surface electrodes to the submental/anterior neck muscles. The only published paediatric study of 95 children receiving a course of 22 sessions (mean) over 10 weeks found no significant difference between NMES compared to usual care with dietary manipulation overall (Christiaanse et al. 2011). Further research is required for all of these interventions.

Texture Modification of Food and Fluids

Modification of fluid consistencies and food textures is commonly recommended to optimise feeding efficiency and swallowing safety for children with oropharyngeal dysphagia. Recommendations for fluid and food textures should be based on a thorough clinical and instrumental evaluation and tailored to the child's specific oral sensorimotor and swallowing skills, feeding efficiency, aspiration risk/safety, fatigue levels and self-feeding independence level by a speech pathologist. The International Dysphagia Diet Standardization Initiative has developed a framework to describe seven levels of fluid/food, with five fluid levels (thin fluids, slightly, mildly, moderately and extremely thick fluids) crossing over five diet levels ranging from liquidised to a regular diet (liquidised, pureed, minced & moist, soft & bite-sized, regular) (Cichero et al. 2017). Different food/fluid consistencies require different levels of oral sensorimotor competency and swallow response. Thin fluids flow quickly and require a prompt swallow response and intact airway closure to prevent aspiration. Thickened fluids, purees, mashed foods and solids are less likely to cause pharyngeal penetration/aspiration (Weir et al. 2011; Steele et al. 2015); however, they are more likely to have associated pharyngeal residue with its own associated aspiration risk (Weir et al. 2009).

A finding of consistent aspiration on a given texture or fluid consistency often results in that consistency being restricted or eliminated from that individual's dietary repertoire. **Thickening fluids** is a common intervention for thin fluid aspiration, with growing evidence to suggest a reduction in laryngeal penetration-aspiration correlates with increasing fluid viscosity (Steele et al. 2015). Care should be taken to thicken fluids only to the extent required to ensure safety, whilst matching the fluid to utensils used to allow appropriate flow rate for safety, efficient intake to meet nutritional requirements, and optimal independence relative to the child's physical function. Infants commonly tolerate 'slightly thick' or 'antiregurgitation' thick fluids through medium- or fast-flow teats whilst maintaining safety and efficiency. If non-drip teats are used with thickened fluids, the infant will need to produce sufficient lip and velopharyngeal closure to achieve adequate suction. Thickened fluids are often used to assist a child to transition from a spout cup to an open cup (e.g. slightly to mildly thick fluids) as the increased viscosity provides increased sensory information and slows the fluid flow, reducing laryngeal penetration-aspiration risk. Liquid medications commonly used with children should be thickened to the prescribed thickness; however, consultation with a pharmacist may be required to check the impact of thickening agents on medication uptake.

When used appropriately, thickeners can assist many children to obtain full fluid requirements orally and reduce aspiration risk (Gosa et al. 2011). Whilst a range of commercial thickeners are available and include thickening agents such as carob bean, xanthan gum, corn or maize starch, care should be taken to determine whether the product can be used with infants with respect to gestational age and gastrointestinal issues as well as those with allergy. Use of carob bean gum thickeners for gastroesoph-ageal reflux in preterm infants led to fatal necrotising enterocolitis in two preterm infants and development of necrotising enterocolitis in a further 15 infants (Gosa et al. 2011). Thus thickeners should not be used in infants aged less than term corrected age, or those with a recent history of necrotising enterocolitis. Natural thickeners such as rice cereal may be used; however, the cereal may clump, obstruct teats, not thicken fluids uniformly and may also provide additional calories if used to thickened full fluid requirements orally.

Modification of food textures can improve feeding safety and efficiency and reduce fatigue levels. Soft and tough chewable foods require fine motor coordination of the oral phase, and coordination with the pharyngeal phase of swallowing and respiration. Children with mild feeding difficulty may often eat a full range of food textures and chewable foods, and may require simple changes such as softer, slow-cooked meats rather than tough chewable meats or soft, bite-sized portions for chewable foods to maintain efficiency.

Children with severe gross motor impairments may have greater impairment of the oral phase of swallowing and greater risk for choking and asphyxiation. Restricting chewable foods and providing pureed, mashed, 'minced & moist' foods can provide the range of food types in a safer and more easily ingested form, whilst reducing choking risk (Croft 1992).

NUTRITIONAL ADEQUACY, FOOD FORTIFICATION AND SUPPLEMENTATION

A diet that includes a wide variety of foods encompassing all of the food groups (cereals and grains, meats and meat alternatives, dairy and dairy alternatives, fruits and vegetables) is key to nutritional adequacy (Evans et al. 2018) but can be difficult to achieve in children with NI. Including protein rich foods three times per day will assist with meeting protein requirements. Meats can be pureed, minced or prepared using methods to ensure a soft texture and alternatives such as eggs, lentils, legumes and ground nuts can be used. Dairy products and other calcium rich alternatives are convenient and simple ways of including high energy and high protein foods. Homemade milk drinks prepared using additional dried milk powders, cream, ice cream, yoghurts and flavourings boost protein and energy content. Fruits and vegetables provide valuable micronutrients and fibre, but are typically low in energy and protein. The energy content of vegetables and fruits can be increased through adding extra fats/oils and protein rich foods. Examples of extra fats and oils that can be added to foods to provide 100kcal are included in Table 9.2. These can significantly increase the total energy content of many meals and snacks and assist with weight gain.

Care should be taken when using these 100kcal boosters. A high reliance on dairy prod-ucts and these high energy additions to foods and fluids may result in displacement of other foods with valuable micronutrient content.

Table 9.2 100kcal boosters for food and fluid fortification

100kcal boosters	Examples of use
15g butter or margarine	Add to meats and vegetables
30mL pouring cream	Add to fruits, breakfast cereals
	Include in milkshakes
20mL double cream	Add to fruits, breakfast cereals
50g mashed avocado	Blend into milkshakes
	Serve with mashed banana
20g ground almond or other nuts	Add to porridge, include in baked goods
30g grated cheese	Stir through mashed vegetables
	Include cheese sauce with main meals
20g peanut butter or other nut spreads	Stir through vegetables for a satay-style flavour
65g egg	As a snack or mashed into vegetables

Micronutrient deficiencies occur in children with NI due to low micronutrient intakes (see Chapter 8) and can be secondary to low energy requirements, a reduced range of foods consumed and high reliance on fluids (Penagini et al. 2015). Dietary intakes of energy, macronutrients and micronutrients should be assessed and compared against estimated requirements for the child's age and sex. Supplementation may be required to ensure intakes are adequate. Numerous commercial supplements are available for oral use. Some can be added to usual foods or fluids to boost intakes of particular nutrients (such as carbohydrate polymers, protein powders, oils, combined carbohydrate and fat supplements, and vitamin and mineral supplements). Protein powders can be used when protein intakes are inadequate and intake cannot be increased sufficiently through the use of foods. Vitamin and mineral supplementation will be required when dietary intakes are inadequate or when micronutrient deficiency is diagnosed (see Chapter 8). Routine supplementation of vitamin D, regardless of dietary intake, has been recommended for all children with physical disabilities at risk of osteoporosis (Ozel et al. 2016). Other milk- or juice-based oral supplements (sip feeds) contribute significant protein and energy in a nutrient dense and convenient way whilst providing additional micronutrients. There are high energy density varieties and fibre containing options depending on the needs of the child. When fortifying foods and fluids using commercial supplements, care must be taken to ensure dietary intakes for nutrients are adequate and that upper limits for individual nutrients are not exceeded (Bell & Samson-Fang 2013).

Enteral Tube Feeding

Enteral tube feeding is indicated for children who have a functioning gastrointestinal tract and are unable to meet their nutritional requirements through oral intake alone.

For children with NI, the need for enteral tube feeding will be highly related to the child's feeding and swallowing function (Fig. 9.1). In circumstances where weight gain or mealtime safety continues to be poor despite a trial of oral nutrition support and the interventions discussed above, adjunctive tube feeding is appropriate. For children with an unsafe swallow on all food and fluid textures and/or with severe undernutrition, enteral tube feeding will be the first treatment option. For these children, a speech pathologist can be consulted to determine the child's safety for oral tastes, and strategies that may be incorporated to encourage oral exploration and sensorimotor input.

ROUTE OF DELIVERY FOR ENTERAL TUBE FEEDING

The choice of route for delivery of tube feeds depends on the anticipated length of time tube feeding is required, gastrointestinal symptoms (gastroesophageal reflux disease [GORD], vomiting), risk of pulmonary aspiration and previous feed tolerance (if relevant). Most often, tubes are inserted via the nasal passage, or through a stoma into the abdominal wall and tube feeds are delivered via the gastric or postpyloric route.

Nasogastric tubes are soft flexible tubes that are inserted into the stomach via the nasal passage for gastric feeding. They are relatively quick to place, do not require a general anaesthetic, and are suitable for short-term (less than six weeks) tube feeding or as a trial run prior to gastrostomy insertion to provide a period of nutritional rehabilitation and determine any issues with feed tolerance (Bell & Samson-Fang 2013). Gastrostomy tubes (e.g. Percutaneous Endoscopic Gastrostomy or low profile button device) require surgical placement directly into the stomach through an opening in the abdominal wall. For children with severe GORD and to minimise risk of aspiration, an antireflux procedure (i.e. fundoplication) may be done at the same time as gastrostomy placement. Nasogastric tubes have higher rates of discomfort and complications (irritation, ulceration and bleeding, particularly of the nasal passage; displacement and blockages) and require more frequent replacement (Romano et al. 2017), thus gastrostomy is usually the preferred route for longer-term tube feeding (see Chapter 10). Both nasogastric and gastrostomy feeds improve nutritional status in children with NI, often accompanied by improved perception of wellbeing (Romano et al. 2017).

For children with severe reflux and vomiting impacting on their ability to gain weight, and those at high risk of aspiration, feeding directly into the jejunum or postpyloric feeding (nasojejunal, gastrojejunal and jejunal) may be considered. Nasojejunal tubes, similar to nasogastric tubes, enter the enteric tract via the nasal passage with the terminal end placed in the jejunum for postpyloric feeding; gastrojejunal tubes are a combination of a gastrostomy with a tube that extends into the jejunum; and jejunal tubes are inserted directly into the jejunum through an opening in the abdominal wall. Since the jejunum is unable to act as a reservoir, jejunal feeds must be given continuously to prevent diarrhoea and dumping syndrome. This, in combination with the high risk of complications, limits the clinical utility of postpyloric feeding (Romano et al. 2017). Where possible, gastric feeding is the preferred route for enteral tube feeding.

ENTERAL TUBE FEEDING REGIMENS

Enteral feeding regimens can be tailored to suit an individual child's and family's needs. Regimens can include bolus feeds, intermittent or continuous feeds, or a combination of these depending on the child's route of enteral access, feed tolerance, oral intake, volume of feed required, daily activities, and family routine and lifestyle (Bell & Samson-Fang 2013; Romano et al. 2017).

Whilst continuous feeding is necessary for children with postpyloric feeding tubes, breaks in feeding can be provided to allow for activities requiring time away from the feeding pump each day. Continuous feeds are often recommended for children with poor feed tolerance/severe GORD, and those with a high risk of pulmonary aspiration, although published data to support this are limited (Romano et al. 2017). Bolus feeding allows a more flexible feeding schedule, allows development of the hunger–satiety cycle to assist with oral feeding, provides greater opportunity for oral intake, and allows more flexibility for other daily activities. For children able to consume food orally, timing bolus feeds after meals provides opportunity for the development of hunger; and where appropriate can allow for flexibility in the size of the bolus feed, dependent on oral intake. For children with higher energy needs and poor feed tolerance, a combination of overnight continuous feeds and daytime bolus feeds may provide the benefits of both types of feeding regimens whilst achieving adequate nutrition.

TYPES OF FEEDS

Formula selection for a child with NI will be dependent on the child's age, energy requirements, need for nutritional rehabilitation or maintenance, gastrointestinal complications (e.g. GORD, constipation) and previous feed tolerance. Standard (1kcal/mL, 4.2kJ/mL) polymeric formulas, with nutrient compositions adapted for different age groups, are suitable; however, because of the high prevalence of constipation in this group, The European Society for Paediatric Gastroenterology, Hepatology and Nutrition have recommended use of an age appropriate, standard polymeric feed with added fibre for children with NI older than 1 year of age (Romano et al. 2017). A high energy density formula (1.5kcal/mL or 6.3kJ/mL) can be used for children with high energy requirements due to high energy expenditure or nutritional rehabilitation, and can also be used for those with poor tolerance of large feed volumes. In these instances, hydration should be carefully monitored (Romano et al. 2017).

Meeting micronutrient requirements for children with low energy needs can be challenging. Low energy density formulas provide a higher micronutrient composition, relative to energy density; however, additional micronutrient supplementation may still be required. Care should be taken to ensure upper limits of individual nutrients are not exceeded.

BLENDED TUBE FEEDS: PROS AND CONS

The use of blended diets as tube feeds involves the preparation of pureed foods, thinned with liquid to a consistency that can be administered through an enteral feeding tube. Largely driven by carers and families, there has been a resurgence of interest in blended tube feeds as alternatives to commercial formula. However, a recent rapid review found little evidence in favour of blended tube feeds, and the risks regarding safety, nutrition and practical issues remain (Coad et al. 2017). There is some limited evidence to support a reduction in diarrhoea in infants (Kolacek et al. 1996). Claims of reduced gagging and retching following fundoplication surgery (Pentiuk et al. 2011) are not supported by controlled trials. Risks include inadequate energy, protein, fluid and micronutrient intakes (Sullivan et al. 2004; Coad et al. 2017) resulting in micronutrient deficiency and inadequate weight gain (Pentiuk et al. 2011; O'Hara 2015). Contamination can occur during feed preparation with increased risks of infection. Blended tube feeds are more viscous than commercially prepared formula and may result in more frequent tube blockages (Sullivan et al. 2004). The balance of evidence remains in favour of commercially prepared formulas utilising a closed enteral feeding system. Commercial formulas are of known nutritional composition, are easily quantifiable and can be administered with confidence that a child will be meeting their nutritional requirements in a safe way. If, when presented with the pros and cons of blended diets as tube feeds, parents/caregivers wish to continue with this method of feeding, caution should be exercised to ensure safety and nutritional adequacy, with regular monitoring to ensure appropriate weight gain and micronutrient status. It is worth noting that the British Dietetic Association do not recommend the use of blended diets and tube feeds; however, more recently, The European Society for Paediatric Gastroenterology, Hepatology and Nutrition have advised caution if they are used (British Dietetic Association 2016; Romano et al. 2017). The British Dietetic Association do recommend that dietitians work in partnership with their patient and carer to ensure that their emotional needs and preferences are taken into account and that an informed decision can be made about the use of blended diets of tube feeds for the child (British Dietetic Association 2016).

TRAINING NEEDS OF CAREGIVERS

Collaboration with caregivers and mealtime support staff is critical for all aspects of mealtime management discussed in this chapter, both oral and enteral nutrition. Working closely with caregivers can assist clinicians in providing meaningful and appropriate strategies that are responsive to both the child and family's needs and capacity. Thorough, multimodal education and training improves knowledge and skills of caregivers and can reduce the incidence of complications (constipation, diarrhoea and abdominal distension) associated with tube feeding (Chang et al. 2015). By encouraging caregivers to understand the underlying rationale for management decisions as well as the risks associated with not following recommendations, uptake and maintenance of strategies may be improved (Dadds et al. 1984; Chadwick et al. 2002). Recommended strategies to ensure competence include step by step guides, education pamphlets, video recordings and personalised demonstrations by clinicians combined with caregiver return demonstration (Chang et al. 2015). For children commencing tube feeds, information and education is required on the following:

- The goals of tube feeding and anticipated duration

- A written individualised feeding regimen

- Care and cleaning of the feeding tube and skin surrounding the tube

- Methods to confirm tube placement (for nasogastric tubes)

- General hygiene to prevent infection

- Preparation of feeds

- Role and use of equipment including pumps, giving sets, syringes, feed containers etc.

- Troubleshooting and management of potential minor complications

- Advice regarding what to do in an emergency, when to contact a health professional

- Telephone contacts for hospital and community staff

- Detailed information about how to obtain ongoing supplies of equipment and feeds

- Information regarding oral care and hygiene

For children able to consume food orally, tangible and routine goals and adaptive equipment are more likely to be maintained by caregivers than general strategies such as pacing and verbal prompts, and as such these should be emphasised (Chadwick et al. 2002). Further, helping caregivers learn to recognise signs and behaviours during their child's mealtime forms a critical foundation for subsequent strategy use and maintenance, and appropriate and timely professional review (Dadds et al. 1984). Parents/caregivers can learn to identify even specific clinical signs, such as those associated with aspiration, if adequate description and training is provided (Benfer et al. 2015). Practical training in the specific mealtime strategies may include modelling by the therapist, rehearsal or roleplay, and parent quizzes. Implementation at home should ideally be supported by therapist phone contact during the week, in addition to regular face to face appointments to provide feedback and troubleshooting (Dadds et al. 1984).

FOLLOW-UP ARRANGEMENTS

Ongoing MDT monitoring and evaluation of nutrition support for children with NI is essential to ensure ongoing safety, to detect and treat any potential complications, to ensure that nutritional requirements are met and nutritional status is adequate, to re-evaluate the goals of nutrition support and to modify interventions appropriately (see Chapter 7).

Adequacy of energy and protein intake can be monitored objectively through assessment of weight gain and linear growth in children with NI. Individual energy prescription should be altered based on the appropriateness of the child's weight gain, taking into account body composition, as well as changing requirements as children get older. Adequacy of micronutrient intake should be assessed through dietary analysis with measurements of serum levels for individual nutrients when dietary intakes are low. Annual assessment of micronutrient status has been recommended (Romano et al. 2017). Supplementation of calcium should be dependent on diet history as serum levels are not indicative of inadequate intake. Monitoring of gastrointestinal function (for constipation/diarrhoea, GORD, feed intolerance) may lead to alterations in formula and diet prescription, changes to feeding regimens, or alterations to medications. For children with feeding tubes, the integrity of the tube needs to be monitored as well as care of the stoma site.

Frequency of monitoring by the MDT will depend on the age of the child, their nutritional status, nutrient deficiencies, feed tolerance issues, oral sensorimotor/swallowing skill and development, and the general level of support that the family requires. For undernourished children on an initial trial of oral nutrition support, follow-up in 1–3 months is appropriate (Romano et al. 2017). Infants and severely malnourished children will require more frequent follow-up. Children who are gaining weight and growing well should be followed up at a minimum of annually (Mascarenhas et al. 2008). Clinical evaluation of feeding and swallowing should occur annually in children with moderate–severe feeding impairment, with instrumental evaluation occurring when the child's feeding/swallowing has changed or growth-related anatomical change of the head and neck has occurred.

REFERENCES

Arvedson JC (1998) Management of pediatric dysphagia. *Otolaryngol Clin North Am* 31: 453–476.

Arvedson JC (2013) Feeding children with cerebral palsy and swallowing difficulties. *Eur J Clin Nutr* 67(Suppl 2): S9–12.

Babbitt RL, Hoch TA, Coe DA et al. (1994) Behavioral assessment and treatment of pediatric feeding disorders. *Dev Behav Pediatr* 15: 278–291.

Bell KL, Samson-Fang L (2013) Nutritional management of children with cerebral palsy. *Eur J Clin Nutr* 67(Suppl 2): S13–16.

Benfer KA, Weir KA, Bell KL, Ware RS, Davies PSW, Boyd RN (2013) Oropharyngeal dysphagia and gross motor skills in children with cerebral palsy. *Pediatrics* e1553–e1562.

Benfer KA, Weir KA, Bell KL, Ware RS, Davies PSW, Boyd RN (2015) Clinical signs suggestive of pharyngeal dysphagia in preschool children with cerebral palsy. *Res Dev Dis* 38: 192–201.

Bisch EM, Logemann JL, Rademaker AL, Kahrilas PJ, Lazarus C (1994) Pharyngeal effects of bolus volume, viscosity, and temperature in patients with dysphagia resulting from neurologic impairment and in normal subjects. *J Speech Lang Hearing Res* 37: 1041–1049.

British Dietic Association (2016) *Policy Statement: Use of Liquidised Food with Enteral Feeding Tubes.* Birmingham: The British Dietetic Association.

Burklow KA, McGrath AM, Kaul A (2002) Management and prevention of feeding problems in young children with prematurity and very low birth weight. *Inf Young Child* 14: 19–30.

Chadwick DD, Joliffe J, Goldbart J (2002) Carer knowledge of dysphagia management strategies. *Int J Lang Comm Dis* 37: 345–357.

Chang SC, Huang CY, Lin CH, Tu SL, Chao MS, Chen MH (2015) The effects of systematic educational interventions about nasogastric tube feeding on caregivers' knowledge and skills and the incidence of feeding complications. *J Clin Nurs* 24: 1567–1575.

Christiaanse ME, Mabe B, Russell G, Simeone TL, Fortunato J, Rubin B (2011) Neuromuscular electrical stimulation is no more effective than usual care for the treatment of primary dysphagia in children. *Pediatr Pulmon* 46: 559–565.

Cichero JA, Lam P, Steele CM et al. (2017) Development of international terminology and definitions for texture-modified foods and thickened fluids used in dysphagia management: the IDDSI framework. *Dysphagia* 32: 293–314.

Coad J, Toft A, Lapwood S et al. (2017) Blended foods for tube-fed children: a safe and realistic option? A rapid review of the evidence. *Arch Dis Child* 102: 274–278.

Craig GM, Scambler G, Spitz L (2003) Why parents of children with neurodevelopmental disabilities requiring gastrostomy feeding need more support. *Dev Med Child Neurol* 45: 183–188.

Croft RD (1992) What consistency of food is best for children with cerebral palsy who cannot chew? *Arch Dis Child* 67: 269–271.

Dadds MR, Sanders MR, Bor B (1984) Training children to eat independently: Evaluation of mealtime management training for parents. *Behav Psych* 12: 356–366.

Evans C, Hutchinson J, Christian MS, Hancock N, Cade JE (2018) Measures of low food variety and poor dietary quality in a cross-sectional study of London school children. *Eur J Clin Nutr* 72(11): 1497–1505.

Gisel EG (1996) Effect of oral sensorimotor treatment on measures of growth and efficiency of eating in the moderately eating-impaired child with cerebral palsy. *Dysphagia* 11: 48–58.

Gisel EG, Tessier MJ, Lapierre G, Seidman E, Drouin E, Filion G (2003) Feeding management of children with severe cerebral palsy and eating impairment: an exploratory study. *Phys Occ Ther Pediatr* 23: 19–44.

Gosa MM, Schooling T, Coleman J (2011) Thickened liquids as a treatment for children with dysphagia and associated adverse effects: A systematic review. *ICAN* 344–350.

Helfrich-Miller KR, Rector KL, Straka JA (1986) Dysphagia: its treatment in the profoundly retarded patient with cerebral palsy. *Arch Phys Med Rehabil* 67: 520–525.

Hulme JB, Poor R, Schulein M, Pezzino J (1983) Perceived behavioral changes observed with adapted seating devices and training programs for multihandicapped, developmentally disabled individuals. *Phys Ther* 63: 204–208.

Hwang Y, Lin C, Coster WJ, Bigsby R, Vergara E (2010) Effectiveness of cheek and jaw support to improve feeding performance of preterm infants. *Am J Occ Ther* 64: 886–894.

Inal O, Serel Arslan S, Demir N, Tunca Yilmaz O, Karaduman A (2017) Effect of Functional Chewing Training on tongue thrust and drooling in children with cerebral palsy: a randomised controlled trial. *J Oral Rehab* 44: 843–849.

Kaviyani Baghbadorani M, Soleymani Z, Dadgar H, Salehi M (2014) The effect of oral sensorimotor stimulations on feeding performance in children with spastic cerebral palsy. *Acta Med Iran* 52: 899–904.

Kolacek S, Grguric J, Percl M, Booth IW (1996) Home-made modular diet versus semi-elemental formula in the treatment of chronic diarrhoea of infancy: a prospective randomized trial. *Eur J Pediatr* 155: 997–1001.

Lanert G, Ekberg O (1995) Positioning improves the oral and pharyngeal swallowing function in children with cerebral palsy. *Acta Paediatrica* 84: 689–692.

Law-Morstatt L, Judd DM, Snyder P, Baier RJ, Dhanireddy R (2003) Pacing as a treatment technique for transitional sucking patterns. *J Perinatol* 23: 483–488.

Logemann JA (1998) *Evaluation and Treatment of Swallowing Disorders.* Austin, TX: PRO-ED.

Mascarenhas MR, Meyers R, Konek S (2008) Outpatient nutrition management of the neurologically impaired child. *Nutr Clin Pract* 23: 597–607.

Mathisen B, Skuse D, Wolke D, Reilly S (1989) Oral-motor dysfunction and failure to thrive among inner-city infants. *Dev Med Child Neurol* 31: 293–302.

Mirrett PL, Riski JE, Glascott J, Johnson V (1994) Videofluoroscopic assessment of dysphagia in children with severe spastic cerebral palsy. *Dysphagia* 9: 174–179.

Morris SE, Klein MD (2000) *Pre-Feeding Skills, Second Edition: A Comprehensive Resource for Mealtime Development.* United States: TSB/Harcourt.

Morton RE, Bonas R, Fourie B, Minford J (1993) Videofluoroscopy in the assessment of feeding disorders of children with neurological problems. *Dev Med Child Neurol* 35: 439–448.

O'Hara C (2015) Scurvy related to the use of a homemade tube feeding formula. *Inf Child Adolesc Nutr* 7: 381–384.

Ozel S, Switzer L, Macintosh A, Fehlings D (2016) Informing evidence-based clinical practice guidelines for children with cerebral palsy at risk of osteoporosis: an update. *Dev Med Child Neurol* 58: 918–923.

Penagini F, Mameli C, Fabiano V, Brunetti D, Dilillo D, Zuccotti GV (2015) Dietary intakes and nutritional issues in neurologically impaired children. *Nutrients* 7: 9400–9415.

Pentiuk S, O'Flaherty T, Santoro K, Willging P, Kaul A (2011) Pureed by gastrostomy tube diet improves gagging and retching in children with fundoplication. *J Parent Enter Nutr* 35: 375–379.

Ptomey LT, Wittenbrook W (2015) Position of the Academy of Nutrition and Dietetics: nutrition services for individuals with intellectual and developmental disabilities and special health care needs. *J Acad Nutr Diet* 115: 593–608.

Reau NR, Sentunce YD, Lelailly SA, Christoffel KK (1996) Infant and toddler feeding patterns and problems: Normative data and a new direction. *J Dev Behav Pediatr* 17: 149–153.

Romano C, Van Wynckel M, Hulst J et al. (2017) European Society for Paediatric Gastroenterology, Hepatology and Nutrition guidelines for the evaluation and treatment of gastrointestinal and nutritional complications in children with neurological impairment. *J Pediatr Gastroent Nutr* 65: 242–264.

Sharp WG, Jaquess DL, Morton JF, Herzinger CV (2010) Pediatric feeding disorders: a quantitative synthesis of treatment outcomes. *Clin Child Fam Psych Rev* 13: 348–365.

Snider L, Majnemer A, Darsaklis V (2011) Feeding interventions for children with cerebral palsy: a review of the evidence. *Phys Occ Ther Pediatr* 31: 58–77.

Stavness C (2006) The effect of positioning for children with cerebral palsy on upper-extremity function. *Phys Occ Ther Pediatr* 26: 39–53.

Steele CM, Alsanei WA, Ayanikalath S et al. (2015) The influence of food texture and liquid consistency modification on swallowing physiology and function: a systematic review. *Dysphagia* 30: 2–26.

Stratten M (1981) Behavioural assessment scale of oral functions in feeding. *Am J Occ Ther* 35: 719–721.

Sullivan MM, Sorreda-Esguerra P, Platon MB et al. (2004) Nutritional analysis of blenderized enteral diets in the Philippines. *Asia Pac J Clin Nutr* 13: 385–391.

Toomey KA, Ross ES (2011) SOS Approach to feeding. *SIG 13 Persp Swall Swall Dis (Dysphagia)* 20: 82–87.

Weir K, McMahon S, Barry L, Masters IB, Chang AB (2009) Clinical signs and symptoms of oropharyngeal aspiration and dysphagia in children. *Eur Resp J* 33: 604–611.

Weir KA, McMahon S, Taylor S, Chang AB (2011) Oropharyngeal aspiration and silent aspiration in children. *Chest* 140: 589–597.

Winstock A (2005) *Eating and Drinking Difficulties in Children: A Guide For Practitioners.* New York: Routledge.

CHAPTER 10

Enteral Tube Feeding: Practical and Ethical Considerations
Peter B Sullivan

INTRODUCTION

Progress in neonatal intensive care techniques have resulted in improved survival of extremely preterm and low-birthweight neonates. Of those that survive from extreme prematurity, 25% will have permanent psychomotor problems including feeding and nutritional problems (Costeloe et al. 2012). Many of these children will grow up with a disability so profound that they are never likely to become independently mobile, to communicate effectively with others or to feed themselves.

At least a third of children with moderate to severe cerebral palsy (CP) will have feeding difficulties. Malnutrition should not be considered normal in children with CP. Early, persistent and severe feeding difficulties are a marker for subsequent poor growth and developmental outcomes. Growth patterns in children with CP are associated with their overall health and social participation. Growth restriction increases progressively with age and thus mandates early nutritional intervention. In children with severe CP such nutritional intervention is increasingly being administered by gastrostomy feeding tube but controversy surrounds the evidence base for this approach. Moreover, parental decisions about gastrostomy feeding are complex and difficult and must be taken into account in making therapeutic recommendations. This chapter discusses the available research evidence and psychosocial issues around gastrostomy feeding in children with severe CP. It seeks to provide a basis for rational clinical decision making based upon the integration of the best available research evidence with clinical experience and patient values.

CONSEQUENCES AND MANAGEMENT OF UNDERNUTRITION

The main consequence of undernutrition is growth failure. Chapter 5 deals with this issue in detail. Children with moderate or severe CP have poor growth compared with typical children and this correlates with markers of health and social participation; well-nourished children with CP have better health and more social participation than similar undernourished children (Liptak et al. 2001; Stevenson et al. 2006).

Enteral Tube Feeding

The principles of nutritional assessment and management are described in the preceding chapters. Enteral tube feeding is frequently indicated in children with CP with significant oropharyngeal incoordination who are unable to meet their nutritional requirements orally.

Nasogastric tube feeding is mostly used for short-term enteral tube feeding – often prior to insertion of gastrostomy tube. There are several limitations for long-term nasogastric tube use, including nasal discomfort, irritation or penetration of the larynx, oesophageal erosion, recurrent pulmonary aspiration, and blockage or displacement of the tube. Weight gain in children followed for over a year is better in those with a gastrostomy compared with those with a nasogastric tube (Samson-Fang et al. 2003). Furthermore, survival rates among children with severe neurological disabilities fed by gastrostomy tube are significantly better than those fed by nasogastric tube.

INDICATIONS FOR GASTROSTOMY TUBE FEEDING

The range of indications for insertion of a gastrostomy feeding tube in paediatrics is extensive. The commonest indication for gastrostomy insertion is to overcome oral motor impairment and feeding difficulties in children with neurological impairment (predominantly CP). Insertion of a gastrostomy feeding tube is an increasingly common intervention in neurologically impaired children who have a clinically unsafe swallow; are unable to maintain a satisfactory nutritional state by oral feeding alone; have an inordinately long (> 3h/day) oral feeding time; and are dependent on nasogastric tube feeding (Sullivan et al. 2005). Nevertheless, children who have a percutaneous endoscopic gastrostomy tube inserted for the treatment of aspiration are twice as likely to be subsequently admitted to hospital than those fed orally; this is largely related to postoperative complication of the procedure (see below) (McSweeney et al. 2016).

METHODS OF INSERTION

For much of the twentieth century the Stamm gastrostomy, which requires surgical laparotomy, was the most commonly accepted insertion technique. The Percutaneous

Endoscopic Gastrostomy (PEG) technique introduced in the 1980s has the advantage that it is minimally invasive, can be performed by a gastroenterologist, is relatively inexpensive and, if the patient's condition precludes use of a general anaesthetic, it can be performed under sedation. PEG tube insertion can be performed as a day case, preferably under general anaesthesia, and takes less than ten minutes. Nevertheless, children are often admitted to hospital for a period postoperatively for monitoring and initiation of feeds.

Shortly following the introduction of PEG, a percutaneous image-guided alternative to surgical and endoscopic gastrostomy placement, the percutaneous gastrojejunostomy (GJ) was introduced. In contrast to the open and PEG approaches, the radiological technique obviates a laparotomy incision or gastroscope, respectively, and is therefore considered the least invasive gastrostomy insertion technique (Ho 1983). Furthermore, image-guided gastrojejunal tubes may be a useful alternative to fundoplication and gastrostomy for neurologically impaired children with gastroesophageal reflux (Wales et al. 2002). Nevertheless, GJ necessitates a continuous feeding regimen, requires additional procedures if the tube becomes dislodged or has to be repositioned, and in rare circumstances can cause a life-threatening intussusception (Livingston et al. 2015). Despite being less invasive, this relatively blind approach has been associated with unique complications including placement of the catheter through a lobe of the liver and fistulation into the small bowel. This technique is not often used in children as the evidence base is so poor although antegrade percutaneous fluoroscopically guided gastrostomy is growing in popularity (Nah et al. 2010).

In 1990, laparoscopic assisted gastrostomy (LAG) placement was introduced, combining the minimally invasive advantages of PEG with the safety of the open procedure allowing for tube placement under direct visualisation. PEG is associated with an increased risk of major complications when compared to the laparoscopic approach. Advantages in operative time appear outweighed by the increased safety profile of laparoscopic gastrostomy insertion (Baker et al. 2015). Hansen (2017) also found that postoperative complications (mostly minor and which occurred in over half of the children in their study) were more common following the pull-through technique than with the laparoscopic approach (Hansen et al. 2017). Nevertheless, a less clear-cut situation emerged from a systematic review and meta-analysis which failed to find sufficient evidence on which to base a firm recommendation on the choice between the PEG and LAG techniques (Suksamanapun et al. 2017).

Skin level 'button' gastrostomy tubes provide an easy and comfortable approach to enteral nutrition. Development of a single-stage percutaneous technique for gastrostomy button insertion rather than the two-stage technique is popular in some centres.

An antireflux procedure (i.e. fundoplication) to decrease risk of aspiration due to gastric reflux may be done simultaneously with surgical gastrostomy although such an approach should not be routine (Langer et al. 1988; Wheatley et al. 1991; Puntis et al. 2000; Kakade et al. 2015; Aumar et al. 2018). Current guidelines and reviews do not provide evidence to support superiority between either fundoplication/gastrostomy (FG) or GJ feeding in children with neurological impairment (NI) who have gastroesophageal reflux disease unresponsive to medical management; the risk of early and late major complications appears to be higher with FG whereas the frequency and burden of tube changes appear to be greater with GJ (Livingston et al. 2015).The gastrostomy tube in a child with a fundoplication can be changed without sedation at home or in clinic, while changing a gastrojejunal tube requires conscious sedation and a procedure in hospital.

BENEFITS OF GASTROSTOMY TUBE FEEDING

In children with NI, gastrostomy placement has been shown to significantly increase weight gain and to be associated with a reduction in all of the following: feeding time, drooling, feed-related choking episodes, vomiting and frequency of chest infections (Rempel et al. 1988; Sullivan et al. 2000, 2005; Samson-Fang et al. 2003; Marchand & Motil 2006; Romano et al. 2017). Malnourished children with severe CP show significant increases in body fat with gastrostomy tube feeding (Sullivan et al. 2006; Vernon-Roberts et al. 2010). Such children have a rapid response to nutritional support through gastros-tomy with catch-up growth regardless of age, even though there is a more pronounced state of malnutrition as age increases. Furthermore, death rates are distinctly higher in the subgroup of children with the most pronounced state of malnutrition and multiple secondary chronic conditions before gastrostomy.

Anecdotal reports in different studies have suggested that early developmental progress, pubertal development and emotional temperament improved following gastrostomy feeding but this needs more detailed research.

Family stress is significantly reduced and quality of life of parents increases after gas-trostomy insertion to assist feeding (Mahant et al. 2009). Parents spend less time on child care once tube feedings are initiated and find feeding less difficult. This leads to evidence of caregiver satisfaction with gastrostomy tube feeding in the majority of studies (Nelson et al. 2015).

COMPLICATIONS OF GASTROSTOMY TUBE FEEDING

It is difficult to make meaningful statements about risks and complications from the published data because types and rates of complications are not reported in a stand-ard way and some children experience multiple complications. Moreover, reports on complications related to PEG are hampered by the lack of consensus regarding the definition of complications and because complications can occur several months after placement. There is, therefore, a need for agreement on the definition of complications related to gastrostomy insertion (Hansen et al. 2017). Insertion of a gastrostomy feeding tube carries with it a relatively low risk of complications. Published literature suggests a procedure-related mortality of 1%, a major complication rate ranging from 6% to 12% and a minor complication rate of at least 50% (Hansen et al. 2017).

Reported major complications of gastrostomy insertion include adverse anaesthetic events, oesophageal laceration, pneumoperitoneum, peritonitis, colonic perforation and cologastric fistula formation. Many of these complications are now avoided or reduced in likelihood by refinements to the technique of insertion.

Later complications include stoma leakage, cellulitis, granulation tissue formation around the gastrostomy site and displacement. Gastrostomy site infection is the commonest problem occurring in up to 20% of cases but is easily and successfully treatable. More serious later complications such as bowel obstructions, gastrointestinal bleeds, ulceration and peritonitis are rare. Other later gastrointestinal complications include constipation, diarrhoea, cramping and vomiting. Although in the majority of cases PEG placement does not induce symptomatic GOR, it may worsen GOR and necessitate the use of antireflux medication or surgery.

Recent evidence suggests that half of children develop delayed gastric emptying after laparoscopic gastrostomy; this increases the risk of postoperative leakage and feeding intolerance and may be associated with GOR (Franken et al. 2017). This study, which was the first prospective study of delayed gastric emptying before and after gastrostomy tube placement, did not however demonstrate a worsening of GOR following gastrostomy tube insertion.

Death rates following gastrostomy range from 14% (after 1 year) to 26% (after 5 years). Most workers concur that these death rates are indicative of the severe morbidity (usually related to chronic secondary conditions including oesophagitis and lung disease from repeated pneumonias) in the children before gastrostomy.

What to Feed with Enteral Tubes

A consideration of what type of feed to use with enteral tubes is beyond the scope of this chapter and has been dealt with in detail in Chapter 9. Suffice to say that against a background of published evidence to support the efficacy of standard polymeric tube feeding for children with NI (Dipasquale et al. 2018), the current topic of debate concerns the use of home blended diets versus proprietary enteral feeds (Breaks et al. 2018). At the present time, authorities recommend caution when use of home blended diets is considered (European Society for Paediatric Gastroenterology, Hepatology and Nutrition; British Dietic Association) as concerns continue over the nutritional adequacy and safety of such diets (Coad et al. 2017; Romano et al. 2017).

Risk of Overfeeding

Immobile children with spastic four limb CP who are exclusively fed by gastrostomy tube grow consistently on an energy intake of less than 7kcal/cm, that is, diets ranging from 500–1100 kcal/day. Remarkably, this intake is 16–50% less than the recommended daily allowance. These extremely low energy intakes often make doctors, nurses and dietitians hesitant to accept the adequacy of such diets. The consequences of this may be overfeeding with the attendant risk of excessive fat storage. Use of high energy proprietary enteral feeds in children with CP fed by gastrostomy tube exacerbates the risk of overfeeding and has a potentially adverse effect on body composition (Sullivan et al. 2006). Conversely, low energy but nutritionally complete enteral feeds can produce weight gain without excess fat deposition (Vernon-Roberts et al. 2010).

Timing of Gastrostomy Insertion

Given what we now know about the benefits of gastrostomy tube feeding, there is a remarkable variation in its application across Europe with usage in over two thirds of children with CP (Gross Motor Function Classification System levels IV–V) in western Sweden but only 12% in such children in Portugal (Dahlseng et al. 2012a). This variation in usage was accompanied by variation in degree of growth retardation with those in Sweden being the least and those in Portugal being the worst affected. There was similar variation found in age at gastrostomy tube placement ranging from 16 months of age in Sweden to 70 months of age in northern England.

As increasing numbers of children with CP are undergoing gastrostomy insertion and are now surviving beyond childhood into adulthood, the question arises as to whether optimum long-term benefit could be achieved by gastrostomy placement at an early stage within this patient group. The evidence from several studies is that attainment of minimum growth standards occurs more frequently in children treated early before malnutrition and morbidity become established (Martinez-Costa et al. 2011; Sharma et al. 2012). Early nutritional supplementation by gastrostomy results in improved linear growth and weight-for-age z-score in children with severe CP if commenced early in life (less than 18 months) (Marchand & Motil 2006). Conversely, morbidity and mortality are most prevalent in those who receive gastrostomy later in life, that is, children treated 8 years or more after central nervous system insult.

Exhaustion with feeding as a neonate and persisting feeding difficulties at 6 months are associated with more severe neurodevelopmental and growth impairments in school age children with CP (Hawdon et al. 2000; Strand et al. 2016; Jadcherla et al. 2017). These observations may help identify those children with CP who may benefit from early assessment and interventions including gastrostomy insertion.

Recent evidence from Norway is that, although the prevalence of gastrostomy tube use there is increasing, only two thirds of children with significant feeding problems are tube fed, which possibly suggests that too few children have this treatment. Dahlseng and colleagues found that children with poor motor and speech function were older at placement of the gastrostomy tube and that the age of placement of a gastrostomy tube had an inverse effect on growth status. Some children have their gastrostomy tube inserted too late to achieve optimal growth and health (Dahlseng et al. 2012b).

Later insertion of gastrostomy may relate to parents' concerns of complications such as reflux-related respiratory illness in the most severely affected children and abhorrence of the idea of gastrostomy feeding (see below). Nevertheless, as noted above, most studies show that that the majority of parents would have agreed to earlier gastrostomy feeding of their children had they acknowledged its benefits.

Parents' Perceptions

Application of a strict biomedical model with emphasis on growth and symptoms is likely to neglect parental concerns about gastrostomy tube feeding. Craig approached this issue from a feminist poststructuralist perspective: she notes 'women are faced with enormous responsibility for making decisions about a child's nutritional management but may feel almost powerless in the face of uncertainty as to whether or not their child will benefit from a gastrostomy tube, and if so, at what cost?' (Craig & Scambler 2006). Such factors can significantly influence quality of life outcomes.

The severity of the disease as well as the presence and severity of malnutrition both have a negative impact on quality of life (QoL). Gastrostomy feeding is effective in reversing malnutrition in children with NI and has positive effects on the QoL of the patients and the caregivers. QoL is often the most important outcome of treatment for chronic conditions such as NI (Bjornson & McLaughlin 2001). Children with NI have reduced health-related QoL and the degree to which it is reduced is related to the severity of their NI (Samson-Fang et al. 2002; Vargus-Adams 2005). Almost 50% of children with NI are able to self-report their perceptions of their health-related QoL. Healthcare professionals and parents should, therefore, rely on a proxy report only when the children are not capable of self-report, or to ascertain potential differences in perceptions between children and their parents (Varni et al. 2005). Nevertheless, for severely disabled children parent-proxy reported QoL are the only available data. Caring for a child with NI affects a parent's physical well-being, social well-being, freedom, independence, family well-being and financial stability (Davis et al. 2012). Carers of children with NI have poor QoL, worse mental health and higher burnout levels than controls (Basaran et al. 2013). Parents often feel unsupported by the services they access (Craig et al. 2003). Children with the most severe motor disability who have feeding tubes are an especially frail group, that is, having the poorest health, the worst well-being and using the most health-related resources (Liptak et al. 2001). Previous qualitative studies have found issues of social isolation, difficulty in obtaining care and high caregiving demands among parents of children with NI who are fed through a gastrostomy tube (Thorne et al. 1997; Craig & Scambler 2006).

Gastrostomy tube placement is often delayed because of negative caregiver perceptions. This delay may occur despite multiple hospital admissions for respiratory infections due to aspiration. Paradoxically, these parents are often less tentative about allowing other more invasive procedures such as orthopaedic surgery.

The decision making process for parents when a gastrostomy is first proposed is characterised by conflict (Mahant et al. 2018, 2011). Multiple negative perceptions may coexist in varying degrees. Despite being a struggle, mothers may view feeding by mouth as an enjoyable activity and an important social process. Mothers may feel guilty about their child's poor growth and may perceive the recommendation that gastrostomy feeding is required as confirmation of failure and a disruption of maternal nurturing and bonding. For some mothers gastrostomy feeding represents a loss of normality and may be seen as a confirmation of the permanence of the disability (Thorne et al. 1997; Petersen et al. 2006; Craig et al. 2006). In addition, the loss of oral feeding may be seen as a denial of a basic or essential human pleasure. Fears about loss of normal eating, dependency on gastrostomy feeds, complications of the procedure and the like can make parents very resistant to the idea of gastrostomy tube feeding and, even if they agree, they may choose to use the gastrostomy only as a last resort.

Nonetheless, the majority of caregivers recognise improvement in the children following placement and show high levels of satisfaction (Brotherton et al. 2007; Åvitsland et al. 2012; Nelson et al. 2015). Importantly, the majority admit that they would have accepted an earlier placement of the gastrostomy tube had they anticipated the overall outcome. Both management of the affected child and family relationships are usually accepted as having improved considerably when the feeding difficulties are ameliorated by gastrostomy insertion.

Using a validated instrument for measurement of QoL, Sullivan et al. (2004) found a significant improvement in the QoL of carers 6 and 12 months after insertion of a gastrostomy feeding tube in children with CP (Sullivan et al. 2004), A clear need for additional support for parents of children with a PEG has been identified that goes beyond simply meeting clinical need. Ongoing medical and psychosocial support is needed after initiation of non-oral feeding and is best provided through the collaborative efforts of the family and a team of professionals (Adams et al. 1999).

Interaction with healthcare professionals in relation to the proposition to introduce gastrostomy tube feeding is, however, often characterised by poor communication, lack of information, paternalism and a lack of caregiver participation in decision making (Brotherton et al. 2007). It is clear from the foregoing that a great deal of sensitivity to the fears and feelings of the parents is required when approaching the subject of gastrostomy tube feeding. Parents need detailed information about gastrostomy feeding and support during decision making without pressure from family and healthcare professionals. Understanding these perceptions will help healthcare workers to develop effective, family-centred, patient appropriate intervention and adherence strategies for gastrostomy fed children with CP. All members of the multidisciplinary team should be well informed about the indications for and advantages and disadvantages of tube feeding so that a consistent message is conveyed to parents.

ETHICAL ISSUES

In an update of an earlier systematic review (Sleigh et al. 2004) which found no evidence of sufficiently high quality to merit inclusion, Sanchez (2016) remarked on the unfortunate fact that no randomised control trials comparing the outcomes of gastrostomy and oral feeding for children with CP were conducted in the 9 years between the publication of two Cochrane Reviews (Gantasala et al. 2013; Sanchez et al. 2016). The practical challenges inherent in conducting randomised control trials in this field are considerable. Sleigh and colleagues point out the potential 'complexity and costs of organizing what would necessarily be a large multi-center RCT with power sufficient to detect moderate-sized trial effects' (Sleigh et al. 2004). Furthermore, there are significant ethical challenges in randomising children to treatment groups when this intervention is already widely provided. This issue is poignant given that providing or withholding the intervention may have a significant impact on participants' growth, health and neurodevelopment and that the intervention may have significant side effects, as outlined above (Samson-Fang et al. 2003; Sullivan et al. 2005; Craig et al. 2006).

PEG feeding for reversing malnutrition in children with NI is a therapeutic intervention and as such is governed by standard ethical rules. The decision on initiation of the treatment is based on the likely net balance between advantages and disadvantages in order to promote the best interest of the individual patient. As is the case in other treatments, informed and educated consent of the parents is an important ethical principle. The parents need to be given detailed information on the benefits, risks and alternatives of the treatment and also, enough time to consider the information in order to make a conscious decision. Healthcare workers need to develop effective, family-centred, patient appropriate adherence strategies for gastrostomy fed children with NI. Furthermore, education and training on gastrostomy feeding, both in hospital and in the community, helps the carers of patients to cope during the transition from oral to gastrostomy feeding while continuing social support is essential in order to improve QoL of carers.

PEG feeding is associated with several complications and is costly. Gastrostomy feeding has been shown to reverse malnutrition (Sullivan et al. 2005) and to reduce the number of feed-related choking episodes, vomiting and chest infections. However, the decision making process for parents is often difficult because of negative caregiver perceptions (Petersen et al. 2006) and the gastrostomy tube placement is often delayed (Mahant et al. 2011). Nonetheless, the majority of caregivers recognise improvement in the children following placement and the majority admit that they would have accepted an earlier placement of the gastrostomy tube if they had anticipated the overall outcome (Petersen et al. 2006; Martinez-Costa et al. 2011).

SUMMARY

Malnutrition should not be considered normal in children with CP. The Nutrition Committee of the Canadian Pediatric Society declared that 'it is unacceptable not to treat undernutrition associated with neurodevelopmental disability' (Canadian Pediatric Society 1994). Nutritional intervention should be provided by a multidisciplinary team of professionals to ensure adequate growth, improve quality of life and optimise functional status. Early intervention, ongoing support and continuing follow-up are necessary to safeguard adequate growth and nutrition. One of the most important decisions to be taken in managing a child with severe CP and feeding difficulties is whether and when to insert a gastrostomy feeding tube.

Samson-Fang et al. critically appraised the effects of gastrostomy feeding in children with CP and concluded that the evidence, although limited, was generally in favour of the intervention (Samson-Fang et al. 2003). However, the review was based on only 10 published studies, largely comprising case series with relatively small samples and without a control (i.e. strength of evidence level IV). A systematic review failed to identify any trials that met the review criteria and concluded that there was continued uncertainty about the effects of gastrostomy (Sleigh & Brocklehurst 2004). Most studies have concentrated on severely affected children and are frequently flawed by a lack of valid and repeatable methods for assessing linear growth and body composition in this population.

Existing studies have focused primarily on the impairment domain measuring surgical and anthropometric outcomes. Evidence from the most comprehensive case series reported improvements on all weight- and growth-related outcomes (weight, head growth, linear growth, arm circumference and skinfold thickness). In fact, all studies to date report significant weight gain after gastrostomy with the implicit comparison being no weight gain without intervention (Ferluga et al. 2014). Some children remain underweight after intervention but given a lack of appropriate reference standards for the CP population, these results should be interpreted cautiously. Few studies have encompassed considerations about the broader health, psychosocial and economic aspects of gastrostomy feeding in children with CP.

Although the hierarchy of research evidence underpinning the use of gastrostomy in children with neurodevelopmental problems may not be strong (Ferluga et al. 2014; Sanchez et al. 2016) it is important to appreciate that one of the central tenets of 'evidenced-based medicine' is that evidence alone is never sufficient to make a clinical decision. A sound clinical decision is based upon the integration of the best available research evidence with clinical experience and patient values. This will involve a trade-off between benefits and risks, inconvenience and costs and the concerns, preferences and expectations of the patient/carer. When these elements are assimilated healthcare professionals and parents of children with CP can form a 'therapeutic alliance' to optimise growth, health and quality of life.

REFERENCES

Adams RA, Gordon C, Spangler AA (1999) Maternal stress in caring for children with feeding disabilities: implications for health care providers. *J Am Diet Assoc* 99: 8–6.

Aumar M, Lalanne A, Guimber D et al. (2018) Influence of percutaneous endoscopic gastrostomy on gastroesophageal reflux disease in children. *J Pediatr* 197: 116–120.

Åvitsland TL, Faugli A, Pripp AH, Malt UF, Bjørnland K, Emblem R (2012) Maternal psychological distress and parenting stress after gastrostomy placement in children. *J Pediatr Gastroent Nutr* 55: 562–566.

Baker L, Beres AL, Baird R (2015) A systematic review and meta-analysis of gastrostomy insertion techniques in children. *J Pediatr Surg* 50: 718–725.

Basaran A, Karadavut KI, Uneri SO, Balbaloglu O, Atasoy N (2013) The effect of having a children with cerebral palsy on quality of life, burn-out, depression and anxiety scores: a comparative study. *Eur J Phys Rehabil Med* 49: 815–822.

Bjornson KF, McLaughlin JF (2001) The measurement of health-related quality of life (HRQL) in children with cerebral palsy. *Eur J Neurol* 8: 183–193.

Breaks A, Smith C, Bloch S, Morgan S (2018) Blended diets for gastrostomy fed children and young people: a scoping review. *J Hum Nutr Diet* 31(5): 634–646.

Brotherton AM, Abbott K, Aggett PJ (2007) The impact of percutaneous endoscopic gastrostomy feeding in children: the parental perspective. *Child Care Health Dev* 33: 539–546.

Canadian Pediatric Society (1994) Undernutrition in children with a neurodevelopmental disability. Nutrition Committee, Canadian Paediatric Society. *Can Med Assoc J* 151: 753–759.

Coad J, Toft A, Lapwood S et al. (2017) Blended foods for tube-fed children: a safe and realistic option? A rapid review of the evidence. *Arch Dis Child* 102: 274–278.

Costeloe KL, Hennessy EM, Haider S, Stacey F, Marlow N, Draper ES (2012) Short term outcomes after extreme preterm birth in England: comparison of two birth cohorts in 1995 and 2006 (the EPICure studies). *BMJ* 345: e7976.

Craig GM, Scambler G, Spitz L (2003) Why parents of children with neurodevelopmental disabilities requiring gastrostomy feeding need more support. *Dev Med Child Neurol* 45: 183–188.

Craig GM, Carr LJ, Cass H et al. (2006) Medical, surgical, and health outcomes of gastrostomy feeding. *Dev Med Child Neurol* 48: 353–360.

Craig GM, Scambler G (2006) Negotiating mothering against the odds: gastrostomy tube feeding, stigma, governmentality and disabled children. *Soc Sci Med* 62: 1115–1125.

Dahlseng MO, Andersen GL, da Graca Andrada M et al. (2012a) Gastrostomy tube feeding of children with cerebral palsy: variation across six European countries. *Dev Med Child Neurol* 54: 938–944.

Dahlseng MO, Finbraten AK, Juliusson PB, Skranes J, Andersen G, Vik T (2012b) Feeding problems, growth and nutritional status in children with cerebral palsy. *Acta Paediatrica* 101: 92–98.

Davis E, MacKinnon A, Waters E (2012) Parent proxy-reported quality of life for children with cerebral palsy: is it related to parental psychosocial distress? *Child Care Health Dev* 38: 553–560.

Dipasquale V, Catena M, Cardile S, Romano C (2018) Standard polymeric formula tube feeding in neurologically impaired children: a five-year retrospective study. *Nutrients* 10: 684.

Ferluga ED, Sathe NA, Krishnaswami S, McPheeters ML (2014) Surgical intervention for feeding and nutrition difficulties in cerebral palsy: a systematic review. *Dev Med Child Neurol* 56: 31–43.

Franken J, Mauritz FA, Stellato RK, van der Zee DC, van Herwaarden Lindeboom MYA (2017) The effect of gastrostomy placement on gastric function in children: a prospective cohort study. *J Gastroint Surg* 21: 1105–1111.

Gantasala S, Sullivan PB, Thomas AG (2013) Gastrostomy feeding versus oral feeding alone for children with cerebral palsy. *Cochrane Database Syst Rev* CD003943.

Hansen E, Qvist N, Rasmussen L, Ellebæk M (2017) Postoperative complications following percutaneous endoscopic gastrostomy are common in children. *Acta Paediatrica* 106: 1165–1169.

Hawdon JM, Beauregard N, Slattery J, Kennedy G (2000) Identification of neonates at risk of developing feeding problems in infancy. *Dev Med Child Neurol* 42: 235–239.

Ho CS (1983) Percutaneous gastrostomy for jejunal feeding. *Radiology* 149: 595–596.

Jadcherla S, Khot T, Moore R, Malkar M, Gulati I, Slaughter J (2017) Feeding methods at discharge predict long-term feeding and neurodevelopmental outcomes in preterm infants referred for gastrostomy evaluation. *J Pediatr* 181: 125–130.e1.

Kakade Me, Coyle D, McDowell DT, Gillick J (2015) Percutaneous endoscopic gastrostomy (PEG) does not worsen vomiting in children. *Pediatr Surg Int* 31: 557–562.

Langer JC, Wesson DE, Ein SH et al. (1988) Feeding gastrostomy in neurologically impaired children : Is an antireflux procedure necessary? *J Pediatr Gastroent Nutr* 7: 837–841.

Liptak GS, O'Donnell M, Conaway M et al. (2001) Health status of children with moderate to severe cerebral palsy. *Dev Med Child Neurol* 43: 364–370.

Livingston MH, Shawyer AC, Rosenbaum PL, Jones SA, Walton JM (2015) Fundoplication and gastrostomy versus percutaneous gastrojejunostomy for gastroesophageal reflux in children with neurologic impairment: a systematic review and meta-analysis. *J Pediatr Surg* 50: 707–714.

Mahant S, Friedman JN, Connolly B, Goia C, MacArther C (2009) Tube feeding and quality of life in children with severe neurological impairment. *Arch Dis Child* 94: 668–673.

Mahant S, Jovcevska V, Cohen E (2011) Decision-making around gastrostomy-feeding in children with neurologic disabilities. *Pediatrics* 127: e1471–1481.

Mahant S, Cohen E, Nelson KE, Rosenbaum P (2018) Decision-making around gastrostomy tube feeding in children with neurologic impairment: Engaging effectively with families. *Paediatr Child Health* 23: 209–213.

Marchand V, Motil K (2006) Nutrition support for neurologically impaired children: a clinical report of the North American Society for Pediatric Gastroenterology, Hepatology, and Nutrition. *J Pediatr Gastroent Nutr* 43: 123–135.

Martinez-Costa C, Borraz S, Benlloch C, Lopez-Saiz A, Sanchiz V, Brines J (2011) Early decision of gastrostomy tube insertion in children with severe developmental disability: a current dilemma. *J Hum Nutr Diet* 24: 115–121.

McSweeney ME, Kerr J, Amirault J, Mithcell PD, Larson K, Rosen R (2016) Oral feeding reduces hospitalizations compared with gastrostomy feeding in infants and children who aspirate. *J Pediatr* 170: 79–84.

Nah SA, Narayanaswamy B, Eaton S et al. (2010) Gastrostomy insertion in children: percutaneous endoscopic or percutaneous image-guided? *J Pediatr Surg* 45: 1153–1158.

Nelson KE, Lacombe-Duncan A, Cohen E et al. (2015) Family experiences with feeding tubes in neurologic impairment: a systematic review. *Pediatrics* 136: e140–e151.

Petersen MC, Kedia S, Davis P, Newman L, Temple C (2006) Eating and feeding are not the same: caregivers' perceptions of gastrostomy feeding for children with cerebral palsy. *Dev Med Child Neurol* 48: 713–717.

Puntis JW, Thwaites R, Abel G, Stringer MD (2000) Children with neurological disorders do not always need fundoplication concomitant with percutaneous endoscopic gastrostomy. *Dev Med Child Neurol* 42: 97–99.

Rempel GR, Colwell SO, Nelson RP (1988) Growth in children with cerebral palsy fed via gastrostomy [see comments]. *Pediatrics* 82: 857–862.

Romano C, van Wynckel M, Hulst J et al. (2017) European Society for Paediatric Gastroenterology, Hepatology and Nutrition guidelines for the evaluation and treatment of gastrointestinal and nutritional complications in children with neurological impairment. *J Pediatr Gastroent Nutr* 65: 242–264.

Samson-Fang L, Fung E, Stallings VA et al. (2002) Relationship of nutritional status to health and societal participation in children with cerebral palsy. *J Pediatr* 141: 637–643.

Samson-Fang L, Butler C, O'Donnell M (2003) Effects of gastrostomy feeding in children with cerebral palsy: an AACPDM evidence report. *Dev Med Child Neurol* 45: 415–426.

Sanchez K, Mei C, Morgan AT (2016) No high-level evidence is available comparing gastrostomy or jejunostomy feeding and oral feeding alone for children with feeding difficulties related to cerebral palsy. *Ev Based Comm Assess Interv* 10: 66–70.

Sharma R, Williams AN, Zaw W (2012) Timing of gastrostomy insertion in children with a neurodisability: a cross-sectional study of early versus late intervention. *BMJ Open* 2.

Sleigh G, Brocklehurst P (2004) Gastrostomy feeding in cerebral palsy: a systematic review. *Arch Dis Child* 89: 534–539.

Sleigh G, Sullivan PB, Thomas AG (2004) Gastrostomy feeding versus oral feeding alone for children with cerebral palsy. *Cochrane Database Syst Rev* CD003943.

Stevenson RD, Conaway M, Chumlea WC et al. (2006) Growth and health in children with moderate-to-severe cerebral palsy. *Pediatrics* 118: 1010–1018.

Strand KM, Dahlseng MO, Lydersen S et al. (2016) Growth during infancy and early childhood in children with cerebral palsy: a population-based study. *Dev Med Child Neurol* 58: 924–930.

Suksamanapun N, Mauritz FA, Franken J, van der Zee DC, van Herwaarden-Lindeboom MYA (2017) Laparoscopic versus percutaneous endoscopic gastrostomy placement in children: results of a systematic review and meta-analysis. *J Min Acc Surg* 13: 81–88.

Sullivan PB, Lambert B, Rose M, Ford-Adams M, Johnson A, Griffiths P (2000) Prevalence and severity of feeding and nutritional problems in children with neurological impairment: Oxford Feeding Study. *Dev Med Child Neurol* 42: 10–80.

Sullivan PB, Juszczak E, Bachlet AM et al. (2004) Impact of gastrostomy tube feeding on the quality of life of carers of children with cerebral palsy. *Dev Med Child Neurol* 46(12): 796–800.

Sullivan PB, Juszczak E, Bachlet AM et al. (2005) Gastrostomy tube feeding in children with cerebral palsy: a prospective, longitudinal study. *Dev Med Child Neurol* 47: 77–85.

Sullivan PB, Alder N, Bachlet AM et al. (2006) Gastrostomy feeding in cerebral palsy: too much of a good thing? *Dev Med Child Neurol* 48: 877–882.

Thorne SE, Radford MJ, Armstrong EA (1997) Long-term gastrostomy in children: caregiver coping. *Gastroenterol Nurs* 20: 46–53.

Vargus-Adams J (2005) Health-related quality of life in childhood cerebral palsy. *Arch Phys Med Rehabil* 86: 940–945.

Varni JW, Burwinkle TM, Sherman SA et al. (2005) Health-related quality of life of children and adolescents with cerebral palsy: hearing the voices of the children. *Dev Med Child Neurol* 47: 592–597.

Vernon-Roberts A, Wells J, Grant H et al. (2010) Gastrostomy feeding in cerebral palsy: enough and no more. *Dev Med Child Neurol* 52: 1099–1105.

Wales PW, Diamond IR, Dutta S et al. (2002) Fundoplication and gastrostomy versus image-guided gastrojejunal tube for enteral feeding in neurologically impaired children with gastroesophageal reflux. *J Pediatr Surg* 37: 407–412.

Wheatley MJ, Wesley JR, Tkach DM, Coran AG (1991) Long-term follow-up of brain-damaged children requiring feeding gastrostomy: should an antireflux procedure always be performed? *J Pediatr Surg* 26: 301–304.

Conclusion

Guro L Andersen

In this volume some of the world's leading experts in the field have contributed their knowledge and expertise. This work is intended to assist those multidisciplinary clinical teams responsible for follow-up and treatment of children with neurodisability by providing an up-to-date handbook to aid their decisions regarding assessment and management in these children.

The handbook is a further elaboration of two previous books (1996 and 2009) published by Mac Keith Press dealing with the challenges of feeding and nutrition in children with neurodisability. Because of growing interest and research in this field during the last decade, it seemed timely to produce an update. Thus, the overall aim of this book has been to produce a practical handbook useful for both clinicians new in the field and those more experienced. Many of the chapters have included case reports to underline the message of the chapters.

The first chapter of the book, 'The Normal Development of Oral Motor Function: Anatomy and Physiology', provides a sound basis for understanding the various forms of oromotor problems and feeding difficulties children with neurodisability may experience.

In Chapter 2, '"When Things Go Wrong": Causes and Assessment of Oral Sensorimotor Dysfunction', Diane Sellers has used the International Classification of Functioning, Disability and Health as a framework to explore possible challenges and deviations from typical development of eating and drinking. She emphasises that 'a child's ability to respond automatically, efficiently and comfortably to eating and drinking experiences will be affected by disturbances to sensory processing which include altered registration of sensory input, excessive or low levels of reaction to sensation, limited sensory discrimination, difficulty integrating information and difficulty planning motor responses.' Some standardised clinical assessment tools and eating and drinking ability scales are listed as well as suggestions for instrumental assessments (videofluoroscopy of swallowing and fibreoptic endoscopic evaluations of swallow) and their advantages and disadvantages. Regarding the instrumental assessments, Dr Sellers concludes that the results of investigations must always be interpreted in the context of the clinical picture and the child's quality of life.

Chapter 3, 'Oral Health and Sialorrhea', confirms that there are no intraoral anomalies unique to children with neurodisabilities. However, challenges with oral health and drooling (sialorrhea) are more common than in the typically developing child. Anterior drooling is visible, may cause skin breakdown, predispose to *Candida* infection and has social implications. On the other hand, posterior drooling is not visible but is associated with more clinically significant morbidity. Dr Laurie Glader recommends using the Teacher Drooling Scale for quantifying anterior drooling while posterior drooling is diagnosed by history taking (asking about cough, gagging, choking and recurrent respiratory infections), by clinical examination and/or by identifying aspiration by fiberoptic nasopharyngoscopy and laryngoscopy. Advice is given on possible therapeutic interventions and pharmacological interventions including anticholinergic medications, glycopyrrolate and/or botulinum toxin injection.

Chapter 4, 'Gastrointestinal Problems in Children with Neurodisability: Causes, Symptoms and Management', gives an overview of the most common gastrointestinal problems encountered in children with neurological impairment. Overall, more than 90% of children with neurodisability have gastrointestinal problems like dysphagia/oropharyngeal dysfunction, gastroesophageal reflux or chronic constipation. Oropharyngeal aspiration is present in almost 70% of the most severely impaired children and may cause severe morbidity, so Ilse Broekaert recommends that oropharyngeal dysfunction should be considered in all children with neurodisability even in the absence of obvious clinical signs and symptoms. To diagnose aspiration, imaging diagnostic techniques should be used, of which the gold standard is videofluoroscopy. Gastroesophageal reflux disease is another very common problem and, as these children may be very fragile, a trial of proton pump inhibitors with careful clinical follow-up is an acceptable management. Upper gastrointestinal endoscopy is the method of choice to evaluate oesophageal damage and lower oesophageal pH studies can quantify the exposure of the oesophageal mucosa to acid. Treatment in children consists of lifestyle changes, pharmacological therapies and surgical treatment but the use of proton pump inhibitor treatment is regarded as the most appropriate and cost-effective means of managing long-term gastroesophageal reflux disease in neurologically impaired children.

Chronic constipation affects up to 70% of children with neurodisability and is generally believed to be the result of both neurological and lifestyle factors. Dietary intake of water and fibre is often below the recommended amount and a number of drugs may adversely affect bowel intestinal transit time. Investigations may include transabdominal ultrasound to assess the rectal filling state, or exceptionally an abdominal radiograph. Treatment should follow the standard for typically developing children.

Chapter 5, 'Consequences of Nutritional Impairment' by Jessie M Hulst, gives an overview of clinical consequences of undernutrition, malnutrition and poor nutritional status due to inadequate nutritional intake such as growth failure, cerebral dysfunction, decreased muscle strength and micronutrient deficiencies. The importance of systematic nutritional assessments for all children with neurodisability to avoid nutritional-related comorbidities is emphasised.

In Chapter 6, 'Assessment of Nutritional State: Growth, Anthropometry and Body Composition', Jane Hardy and Hayley Kuter provide an outline of different anthropometric measures relevant for children with neurodisability. In general, they state that weight cannot be used in isolation to assess nutritional status and they emphasise the need for body composition assessment in this group of children.

In Chapter 7, 'Assessment of Nutritional State: Dietetic, Energy and Macronutrients', Kristie Bell and Jacqueline Walker describe possible methods of dietary assessment including the advantages, disadvantages and validity of use in children with neurodisability as well as the clinical utility of each method. They conclude that there is no one method that will assess dietary intake accurately and that the choice of method will depend on the purpose of the dietary intake assessment, the setting and the ability of the parents/carers to be involved. The chapter also includes recommendations on how to estimate energy requirements which are generally lower than in typically developing children while macronutrient, micronutrient and fluid requirements should be based on recommendations for typically developing children and adjusted as required.

In Chapter 8, 'Assessment of Nutritional State: Micronutrient Deficiencies and Bone Health', Steven Bachrach and Heidi Kecskemethy include specific recommendations on how to assess, diagnose and treat compromised bone health in individuals with neurodisability. In children with neurodisability the combination of atypical muscle tone combined with lack of weight bearing results in reduced bone density. It is thus important to ensure sufficient dietary intake of calcium, phosphorus and vitamin D. While adults are treated with a number of different medications and the decision is based solely on the results of bone density assessments, children are sometimes treated for low bone density alone, while others are treated only after a fragility fracture has occurred. Ensuring adequate intake of vitamin D and calcium is essential to help reduce the incidence of fragility fractures but often bisphosphonates are indicated in the treatment of osteopenia/osteoporosis in children with cerebral palsy.

In Chapter 9, 'Feeding and Nutritional Management Strategies', Kristie Bell, Katherine Benfer and Kelly Weir strongly recommend that multidisciplinary teams are needed to evaluate and plan treatment and interventions of nutritional challenges in children with neurodisability. Examples of interventions include correction of micronutrient deficiencies, initiating complete enteral tube feeding, support of mealtime environment and positioning, alterations to food/fluid textures and nutrient density, use of adaptive equipment, caregiver techniques and sensorimotor therapy. In addition, this chapter includes a comprehensive list of possible feeding utensils to provide nutrition safely and efficiently as well as to assist in the development of feeding and swallowing skills.

Chapter 10, 'Enteral Tube Feeding: Practical and Ethical Considerations', starts by stating that although at least a third of children with moderate to severe cerebral palsy will have feeding difficulties, malnutrition should not be considered normal in any child with cerebral palsy. The chapter gives an overview of indications of gastrostomy, methods of insertion, complications, benefits and some considerations about timing of insertion. The chapter also includes ethical considerations regarding the difficult decision parents are required to face when deciding whether or not their child should have a gastrostomy. An important point to remember is that most studies show that the majority of parents would have agreed to earlier gastrostomy feeding of their children had they been fully aware of its potential benefits. The great majority of studies to date report significant weight gain after gastrostomy with the obvious corollary that there is little or no weight gain in undernourished children with cerebral palsy without intervention.

Index

NOTE: Figures and tables are denoted with a lower case, italicised f or t respectively and then their number. (ie. 1f1.1)